Good Food for a Sober Life

Jack Mumey and Anne S. Hatcher, Ed.D., R.D.

CONTEMPORARY
BOOKS, INC.
CHICAGO • NEW YORK

Library of Congress Cataloging-in-Publication Data

Mumey, Jack.
    Good food for a sober life.

    1. Alcoholics—Nutrition.   2. Alcoholism—Diet therapy.
I. Hatcher, Anne S.   II. Title.
RC565.M83   1987   616.86'1063   87-22245
ISBN 0-8092-4804-2

Published by Contemporary Books, Inc.
180 North Michigan Avenue, Chicago, Illinois 60601
Manufactured in the United States of America
Library of Congress Catalog Card Number: 87-22245
International Standard Book Number: 0-8092-4804-2

Published simultaneously in Canada by Beaverbooks, Ltd.
195 Allstate Parkway, Valleywood Business Park
Markham, Ontario L3R 4T8 Canada

Contents

Acknowledgments

The authors are grateful to many people who gave us encouragement and guidance in the creation of this book. It goes beyond the mention of names, for so many people have to give up daily contact with those who set out to lose themselves in the process of writing! Thus, our respective families and colleagues deserve special mention for their patience and support.

Shari Lesser, Contemporary's executive editor, has nurtured this project from the beginning with her own very special way of guidance that makes masses of pages fall into place where chaos has been the rule. Her assistant, Susan Buntrock, has spent many hours poring over the manuscript and organizing it—no small chore!

The authors would not have been able to coordinate chapters if Cynthia Tinsley had not spent many hours running copy and changes back and forth between our two households and offices, a thankless but very necessary task in a project of this kind.

Finally, our thanks to Dr. Steve Carmel for his thoughtful foreword and the hours spent in reading our material to make his comments possible.

Since both of us maintain very busy professional and personal schedules, it seemed that the words of Edna St. Vincent Millay might bring these last few months into focus:

> *My candle burns at both ends;*
> *it will not last the night;*
> *But, ah, my foes, and oh, my friends—*
> *it gives a lovely light!*
> "A Few Figs from Thistles" (1920)

Jack Mumey
Anne Hatcher
January 1987

Introduction

There are probably no other areas in the field of medicine where more controversy exists than in our scientific notions regarding nutrition and chemical dependency. Our ideas are often clouded with misinformation and prejudice. In recent years, however, our knowledge has been expanded and refined. Education still remains the prime agent in clarifying the public's general lack of knowledge in these areas.

The authors of this book have made a wonderful attempt—successfully, I think—at digesting and clarifying some basic facts about nutrition and its relationship to the disease of alcoholism.

As we all know, the delicate human machine requires fuel in order for it to function. This fuel, alias food, must be well balanced with regard to its constituents. Unfortunately, proper nutrition with today's stressful lifestyle is often difficult. Those people in our society who use alcohol to help manage the stress, and sedate their brains, find in time that there are many consequences of that action. This includes not only the toxicity from the alcohol itself but also the results of associated poor nutrition.

The absence of good nutrition is a "death-defying act" all by itself. When coupled with another deadly illness, as it often is, the consequences are usually disastrous. One must therefore learn *recovery* from these sicknesses. Proper education, again, remains our greatest tool. It is therefore imperative that any recovery process includes the reestablishment of good nutritional care. This book clearly defines what those nutritional needs are and how they can be simply managed. This nutritional management must be coupled with anyone's recovery program from alcohol abuse in order for it to be successful.

The authors of this book have made a giant step toward simplifying this complex matter. The recovering person (and I suspect we are all recovering from something), as well as those helping people in recovery, will find this book most helpful.

Stephen Paul Carmel, M.D.

PART I:
NUTRITION
AND THE
RECOVERING
ALCOHOLIC

1
Why Do People Drink?

When Gunthor the caveman would return to his family dwelling after a hard day of battling the saber-toothed tiger or perhaps just driving away other human predators from the entrance to his home, he needed refreshment.

As his mate stirred the fire, Gunthor would pour himself the wonderful liquid that had been sitting, fermenting, in a crude earthenware vessel. The liquid was made from overripe fruits. As Gunthor drank, the cares of the day would slip away. And why not? Gunthor was having a prehistoric "belt or two."

Just like today's drinkers, our Gunthor was receiving some sedation that seemed to dissolve the cares and troubles of the day, at least temporarily. In the Old Testament we find the first recorded instance of drunkenness, when in Genesis 9:20 we read: "Noah was the first tiller of the soil. He planted a vineyard, and he drank of the wine, and became drunk, and lay uncovered in his tent."

2

Today, alcohol is our bestselling tranquilizer, sedative, and general all-around antidepressant. It is also the most abused legal drug available and the drug likely to cause us the greatest amount of permanent physiological damage, not to mention the mind-altering behaviors that we may loosely label as "drunkenness." Alcoholism, as a disease, is also one of the chief causes of vitamin deficiencies, even where there are adequate food supplies.

What happens to us when we drink? What are the changes that occur in our bodies when we get just a "slight buzz"? When we go in for the "hammering" kind of drinking that is going to lead to being totally and completely drunk?

In this chapter, we are going to offer you a look at the effects of alcohol on the body, in the hopes that as you learn more about what alcohol does to destroy, you will be less apt to want to invite that destroyer into your cave!

ALCOHOL AND YOUR BODY

When anyone, not just the alcoholic, takes a drink, the alcohol is absorbed directly into the bloodstream from the stomach, requiring no breakdown as do other foods or liquids. Absorption into the bloodstream is slowed down if any high-fat foods are present in your digestive system. Notice we say "slowed down," not stopped.

Because of this "high-fat braking," bartenders, hosts, and hostesses worldwide serve potato chips, beer nuts, high-fat cheeses, and the like to slow down the alcohol. If you consume these foods you can drink more before feeling the effects of alcohol. The bar will sell more drinks, and you will be able to "handle" your drinks better than your buddy who is trying to drink you under the table!

Add plain water to your drink and the process of

absorption is slowed down even more, due to the dilu-
tion. Add carbonated mixers, though, and the process is
accelerated, because the mixer moves the alcohol
quickly through the stomach to the small intestine,
where absorption into the bloodstream is rapid.

Once the alcohol enters the bloodstream, it goes
almost immediately to the liver, where the process of
detoxification begins. It used to be believed that a good
diet and large amounts of nutritional supplements
could prevent liver damage from alcohol abuse. This is
patently not true. The fact is that liver damage occurs
as a result of alcohol consumption, and no amount of
nutritional precautions will prevent the damage. In
other words, whoever may be telling you, "Eat right,
take your vitamins, then you can drink all you want
without doing any damage to your body," probably is
more of a "saber-toothed tiger" in your life than Gunthor's was! The nutritional problems that result from
alcoholism—and there are many—cannot be relieved
until and unless you stop drinking.

There is no organ in our bodies capable of storing
alcohol until it can be processed, and it certainly is not
as easily eliminated from the body as other wastes are.
When you are constantly running to the bathroom
during your drinking sprees, the need to urinate more
frequently is due more to alcohol's suppression of a
hormone that helps the body retain water than to any
built-in ability of the body to rid itself of alcohol
through urination.

So the alcohol you are consuming is running around
in your bloodstream, waiting for the liver to process it.
Now we need to know how your size and sex affect this
business. The rule is, the larger you are, the more body
fluid you have, hence the lower your blood-alcohol level
and the more alcohol you can consume before it affects
you.

Women have higher percentages of body fat than
men, so they tend to get "higher" on smaller amounts of

alcohol than most men do. Why? Because as the percentage of body fat increases, the level of body fluid drops and so does one's tolerance for alcohol. Since increased body fat and decreased body fluid levels are a normal part of aging, it becomes easy to understand one of the reasons that alcohol tolerance diminishes as we get older.

Now get this: Alcohol is a toxin that affects every cell in your body, a poison that you willingly ingest! It is especially damaging to the liver, the stomach, small intestine, pancreas, adrenal glands, brain, and nerve pathways. How's *that* for destructive!

Look at it this way: all of these organs play vital roles in processing and storing the nutrients obtained from food, nutrients that we all need for daily life. But when alcohol is introduced, all else must be put aside so that the body can begin dealing with this enemy that has invaded the system. Changing the toxic alcohol into a nontoxic form takes priority over every other digestive process. When alcohol is present, vitamins and minerals are poorly absorbed and underutilized. An alcoholic, therefore, is likely to be poorly nourished even if his or her diet contains every essential and nonessential nutrient known to man.

Here's how alcohol affects body organs. Alcohol irritates mucous membranes, especially in the esophagus, stomach, and small intestine. In the stomach, alcohol causes an increased flow of acid and disrupts the protective mucous layer, allowing the acid to attack the lining and possibly produce an ulcer.

Alcohol disrupts digestive enzymes that act on carbohydrates, proteins, and fats, which are normally changed into substances needed by our bodies. Are you a "junk-food" person? Well, alcohol is the number one junk food. It provides nothing in the way of nutrients; it provides only unneeded and unwanted calories. In other words, there is no redeeming value in the use of alcohol from a strictly nutritional standpoint.

The brain is affected, as we all know, by alcohol use. Our brains depend upon glucose (the sugar formed when complex carbohydrates and sugars are digested) in order to function properly. Here's how it works. You start to drink alcohol, and your blood-sugar levels rise for about an hour afterwards. You feel sharper, brighter, wittier, etc., all the behaviors normally associated with "getting high."

Several hours later when blood-sugar levels drop to normal or below, you begin to enter the "mood-swing cycle." Unexplained anger, depression, sleepiness, and poor concentration are some of the behaviors that characterize this stage. You're just not "thinking straight," because of this drop in blood sugar, combined with the reaction to the energy you expended when you started drinking and your blood-sugar levels were high.

Let's move on to the pancreas. This organ releases enzymes specifically designed to change each type of starch or sugar into glucose. One of these enzymes, lactase, is most often affected by alcohol. Lactase helps digest milk sugars, the kind found in milk and ice cream. So once again we see alcohol interfering with a vital digestive process.

This interference occurs in many situations: the conversion of glucose into glycogen (body starch), for example. This conversion process enables our bodies to store energy to be used during times of fasting, such as at night when no food is eaten for almost 12 hours. When alcohol is consumed, the formation of this glycogen is discontinued until the alcohol is cleared from the system.

Well, when the glucose isn't being converted into starch, the body uses it to form fat, and that, folks, adds lots and lots of unwanted pounds, a good example of which is the "beer belly."

Alcohol sends "double messages" to our bodies. Take adrenaline, for example. Adrenaline, the hormone that helps us respond in "fight or flight" situations, is released when we drink alcohol. It raises the blood-sugar level in preparation for dealing with stress.

At the same time that we are getting this increase in blood sugar, insulin is being released to decrease those levels and to keep us feeling "normal." So here's the double message issued by the alcohol: "Drink me. Release adrenaline. *Increase* blood-sugar level." "No! Release insulin. *Lower* blood-sugar levels!" Result? Mood swings leading to poor concentration, possible faintness, or a cold sweat. All of this because blood-sugar levels are fluctuating in an abnormal and "alcohol-forced" manner.

Now for all of you who are familiar with the concepts of "exercise," "aerobics," "training," "pumping iron," and similar activities of the eighties, we're going to let you in on a big fact of "dietary life." It is easier to make fat than to make muscle. Do you know why it is easier to acquire a beer belly than a "man of iron" physique? You see, protein is the substance of which our bodies are made. When alcohol is consumed, enzymes that digest proteins are altered. Since the proteins cannot be used for their intended purpose (building muscle, for example), the amino acids of which they are composed may be converted to fat. So, in place of nice, toned abdominal muscle, we may see our old friend, the beer belly.

Alcohol does something else to amino acids (just in case all this destruction we just talked about isn't enough). Alcohol interferes with the transportation system that gets amino acids to the brain. This in turn interferes with the production of the chemicals in the brain (neurotransmitters) that transmit signals. No wonder people who are drinking begin to transpose thoughts, phrases, words, places, dates, and facts into drunken gibberish! Bad stuff, that booze!

Does any good come to our bodies from drinking alcohol? Well, yes, to a certain extent, assuming you are in the social-drinker category and not an identified alcoholic. Alcohol is considered to be effective in preventing heart disease if one consumes *only* 2½ ounces a day. Small amounts of alcohol seem to raise blood levels of the good kind of cholesterol (called HDL, or high-density lipoproteins), which helps to fight off heart disease.

Of course, when the alcohol drinking gets out of hand, then the reverse happens. Larger amounts of alcohol drunk on a daily basis may cause chest pains (angina), irregular heartbeat (arrhythmia), and other symptoms associated with heart disease.

You know, it's surprising that we don't see more physical signs of malnutrition among recovering people. Not only does alcohol interfere with digestive enzymes, but it also messes up the functioning of the intestinal bacteria and yeasts that aid in digestion. As if that weren't enough, these same intestinal flora, as they are called, produce some of our daily requirement of vitamin B. So alcohol interferes with this process also. No wonder, then, the chances for malnutrition are high as a result of drinking. Look at this:

Fat-soluble vitamins A, D, E, and K may not be absorbed into the bloodstream due to alcohol's interfering with the digestion of fat or the body's inability to convert them into the forms needed to provide nourishment.

Alcohol makes us lose water, so we call it a diuretic. When large amounts of water are lost, so are the water-soluble vitamins, such as vitamin C and the vitamin B complex. Why do we lose the water in the first place? Because alcohol interferes with a hormone whose primary role is to keep the right amount of water in the body. So, when you drink alcohol, you're "throwing out the baby with the bath water."

Alcohol has a greater effect on some vitamins and minerals than on others. Here are some of the highlights:

Vitamin A is itself an alcohol and depends on an enzyme that detoxifies alcohol to be converted into the form in which the body stores and uses it. Our best sources of vitamin A are dark green and dark yellow fruits and vegetables, such as broccoli, spinach, carrots, peaches, and apricots.

Even if we have been eating plenty of these vitamin A–rich foods, our bodies can't use it if alcohol is present. So we begin to see symptoms such as night blindness, blurred vision, and frequent infections as a result of suppressing vitamin A with alcohol. Eating carrots to improve your vision won't do you much good if you are washing them down with alcohol!

Vitamin D is the "sunshine" vitamin. It is essential for the absorption of calcium, phosphorus, and magnesium, and for strong bones and teeth. When we drink alcohol, this vitamin seems not to be as efficiently absorbed by our bodies, and we may even see some garbled messages being transmitted to our nerves and muscles. We may experience irregular heartbeat and real muscle pain. Fortified milk, not alcohol, is a good source of Vitamin D.

The *B-complex vitamins* convert carbohydrates into energy by acting as enzymes. But when alcohol is present in the body, all these vitamins—B_1 (thiamine), B_2 (riboflavin), niacin, B_6, and B_{12}—are used to detoxify the alcohol and therefore are not available for use in other places. What a waste!

Since the B vitamins are all water-soluble to boot, large amounts of them are lost due to the diuretic effect of the alcohol that we described earlier. Three of these vitamins—thiamine, riboflavin, and niacin—are particularly important in detoxifying alcohol, and the body's supplies of these vitamins can be depleted fairly rapidly through the chronic (long-term) use of alcohol.

We need these vitamins. They're important in maintaining the health of nerves and eyes. They promote a sense of well-being, something we all need.

Vitamins B_6 and B_{12} and folate (another B vitamin) play prominent roles in the production of red blood cells, in addition to acting as enzymes in energy production. Alcohol disrupts a protein in the stomach that is necessary for vitamin B_{12} to be absorbed. Some of the breakdown products from alcohol destroy vitamin B_6 and folate, resulting in yet other deficiencies.

Vitamin C is a water-soluble vitamin that helps our bodies produce a substance called collagen. Collagen is a glue that holds us together. When we hear about bleeding gums, aching joints, easy bruising, frequent infections, depression, and just plain "not feeling good," we know there is a vitamin C deficiency lurking about.

Once again, the diuretic effect of alcohol causes the loss of vitamin C in the urine. Alcohol may also cause a disruption of the mucous membranes, which in turn prevents the absorption and use of the vitamin C. Oranges, grapefruit, tomatoes, raw sweet peppers, raw or slightly cooked cabbage, broccoli, cauliflower, brussels sprouts, baked potatoes, and even roasted green chilies are all great sources of this precious vitamin.

Minerals: All minerals are water-soluble, so when we drink alcohol and lose extra water, we lose essential zinc, magnesium, potassium, and calcium from our bodies. More of these minerals vanish if vomiting or diarrhea occurs. These minerals are important for muscle control and nerve transmission, in addition to building strong bones and teeth. Deficiencies of these minerals can cause irregular heartbeat as well as muscle cramps and spasms. The main sources of calcium are milk, yogurt, and cheese. Magnesium comes to us via whole grains, meat, poultry, fish, eggs, and dairy foods. Bananas along with other fruits, are especially high in potassium.

Another mineral, zinc, is needed for eyesight, healing of wounds, the senses of taste and smell, and the production of sperm. When alcohol is present, this zinc must be used by at least 92 enzymes that are pressed

into action to detoxify the alcohol. The recovering
alcoholic may very well exhibit poor wound healing,
poor senses of taste and smell, along with night blindness or blurred vision—all as a result of alcohol abuse
and the subsequent loss of zinc. We look to meat, fish,
poultry, eggs, milk, and cheese for our main sources of
zinc.

Let's recap some of the nutrition-related symptoms
usually found among recovering people. Frequent infections of skin, eyes, kidney, and respiratory system,
poor wound healing, irregular heartbeat, bone loss,
muscle cramps and/or spasms, poor digestion or digestive upsets are common. Low blood count, which can
cause fatigue and shortness of breath (symptoms similar to those of low blood sugar, or hypoglycemia) is
also common. Not enough? How about night blindness,
blurred vision, a poor sense of taste and smell, and
insomnia. Finally, every person who lives with an alcoholic tells us, "He/she has such violent mood swings . . .
he/she is so irritable!"

These are some of the main points about the use of
alcohol and its damage to these marvelous machines we
know as our bodies. Is there hope? Well, of course! The
obvious answer is to get the alcohol out of your life once
and for all and begin the road to recovery. For most
recovering persons, eating regular meals that include a
wide variety of foods will correct most nutrient deficits
over a period of time.

Adding low-potency vitamin and mineral supplements to your diet seems to be helpful. Don't be one of
those persons in recovery who are obsessed with the
idea that they will become dependent on any substance
they ingest.

There's a vast difference between drinking alcohol
and supplementing the diet with necessary vitamins,
minerals, and nutrients that may have been severely
depleted or eliminated through the use and abuse of
alcohol.

As with all the information that we are giving you in this book, you will have the opportunity to evaluate the usefulness of the foregoing descriptions to your own personal program of recovery. What you can use, use. What does not seem to work for you, feel free to discard. The important point to remember throughout this book is that giving up the alcohol is the first and in many ways the easiest (although you may not think so) step in a total program of recovery.

If our hypothetical caveman Gunthor returned one day to find his secure cave devastated by beasts or earthquake, he would have only two choices. Abandon the cave and seek a new one, or rebuild the old one and restore the things that were lost. Your body is that cave, and since we assume you are not willing to die before your time, you are left with the challenge of rebuilding, nourishing, and strengthening the precious gift of life that is yours.

2
Popular Nutritional Theories of Alcoholism

It would really be easy, not to mention convenient, if we could tell you that there is just one universally accepted theory about the cause of alcoholism. Unfortunately, there are many factors that combine in an individual to produce alcoholism; genetic, environmental, physical, and psychological factors are all interwoven in this disease.

In discussing nutrition's impact on alcoholism we have selected a few of the most popular theories for your consideration, with this special admonition: the real reasons for drinking alcohol to excess or becoming addicted to alcohol are as varied as the personalities and body types of the individuals themselves.

So, let's look at these theories. You have probably read about them or seen them cropping up from time to time as researchers uncover more data about alcoholism.

We haven't come so far in history that yesterday's "snake oil" salesmen have completely vanished from the scene. There are plenty of them still around to take your bucks, as they expound on "a sure cure for alcoholism."

Such a cure does not exist. There is no one treatment for alcoholism, be it in the form of a diet or a pill. Each of us is unique; what works well for one person may or may not work well for another. As long as we have alcoholics in the world, we will be exposed to new theories, each one promising to be the *only* or the *best* treatment for alcoholism. *Caveat emptor:* Let the buyer beware.

THE GENOTROPIC THEORY

This theory was advanced in 1970 by the noted biochemist and nutritionist, Dr. Roger Williams. His thesis is that alcoholism is the result of genetic traits and nutritional intake. In his book, *Alcoholism: the Nutritional Approach*, he states that some persons have a need for larger amounts of specific nutrients than others. And he believes that when these needs are not met, and the person consumes alcohol, the concentration of these nutrients in the person's diet is diluted, leading to greater nutritional deficiencies.

Dr. Williams also believes that alcohol weakens the regulatory centers of the brain, especially those that regulate appetite and our control of what we eat and drink. Because of these factors, Dr. Williams theorizes, a person is compelled to drink alcohol and no amount of knowledge or *will power* can counteract the urge to drink.

Williams based his theory on studies he conducted with laboratory rats. He noted that diet-deficient rats preferred alcohol to water, while the opposite was true of rats whose diets were nutritionally adequate. By experimenting with these animals, Williams discovered that if he supplemented the diets of the rats with vitamin B complex, the result was decreased alcohol consumption.

The response from alcoholics who followed Williams's guidelines for reducing sugar intake, consuming food from all the basic food groups, and taking supplements, was positive. They wrote to him saying that by doing these things they had eliminated their desire for alcohol. In later editions of his book, Dr. Williams reported that supplementing the diet with an amino acid known as glutamine, even without the alcoholic's knowledge, seemed to remove the desire for alcohol.

A leading pharmaceutical company even produced and marketed a multivitamin and mineral supplement, using the guidelines established by Dr. Williams. The Williams theory has some basis in fact. Alcoholics do seem to be genetically different from the rest of the population.

In addition to whatever genetic factors are at work in producing alcoholism, part of the difference also seems to stem from different nutritional needs. Dr. Williams's theory that each of us is different biochemically is well established, since each human body is unique in its organ structure and chemical composition.

With the exception of identical twins, no two of us is alike, even though we may have many common features. It stands to reason, then, that each of us has different nutritional needs, and that the amount of a specific vitamin or mineral needed by one person may not be the same as that required by another.

It is "entirely logical," as the fabled Mr. Spock of "Star Trek" might say, that (1) the bodies of persons likely to become addicted to alcohol are different from those of persons who do not drink compulsively; and therefore, (2) the nutritional needs of alcoholics are also different.

Unfortunately, no exact figures are available as to what these differences are. Many research studies have been conducted to confirm this genotropic theory of alcoholism. In typical studies, alcoholics were given instructions on what and how to eat, along with supplements, while a control group of alcoholics was given none.

After 6 to 12 months of following these groups, it was reported that those alcoholics who had the dietary instruction and supplements showed a lower relapse rate. Here may be the first "fly in the ointment" of this theory. Many people (including the authors) who work in the field of alcohol therapy believe that three years is a more realistic time period to follow such groups of alcoholics to see if they "relapse"—return to drinking alcohol on a regular basis.

The second problem arises in the reporting of results themselves. Unless subjects of the study are under close clinical supervision, such as in a hospital, how do you control their food intake and diet supplements? In other words, how do you know that everyone is really sticking to the plan? When you take into consideration that the conclusions were based on self-reported data and that the subjects reported what they ate based on their memories of the previous 24 hours, then the entire theory is called into question. Why? Because the typical alcoholic will often tell us what he or she thinks we want to know, instead of what might really have happened.

When the Williams theory about the use of the amino acid glutamine captured the public's fancy, trouble began to cloud the bright horizon. Supplements of this amino acid are sold in some health-food stores and pharmacies as cures or preventative treatment for alcoholism. They are easily obtained because no prescription is required.

But within the last few months, some adverse medical reactions have been reported. For example, the Tufts University Nutrition Letter of May 1986 reported on two patients who had been taking up to 4 grams of glutamine for a short time. They observed symptoms in these patients that included insomnia, delusions of grandeur, and uncontrolled sex drive.

While the last symptom may seem like a great thing at first sight it truly is not. Fortunately, all of these symptoms disappeared after a few days of abstinence from glutamine. On the positive side of Dr. Williams's theory is the emphasis on a diet high in nutrition and the use of low levels of the nutrients most likely to be affected by excessive drinking. This is particularly important because, at the time of the publication, the effects of alcohol on zinc, magnesium, potassium, and other minerals were not well established.

THE THIQ MODIFICATION THEORY

Here is a widely used and much discussed theory that deals with the chemical changes that occur in the brain when alcohol is present. To help you understand this theory, we need to do a little imagining.

In our bodies there are specific places—"receptor sites"—to which individual chemicals or nutrients must attach themselves in order to cause the desired reaction. These receptor sites are found primarily in two places: (1) in the lining of the small intestine, and (2) in the brain. The small intestine receptor sites are where the vitamins, minerals, and building blocks of protein (amino acids) are absorbed. In the brain, we find the specialized chemicals that cause us to sleep, wake up, feel "high," relax, and even process new information, such as we hope you are doing now.

So these receptor sites are very important to how we live. Let's explore a little deeper into our brains. We have a brain chemical called *enkephalin*, which acts in much the same manner as morphine. For example, when you are in pain or you do something that has the potential of producing pain such as distance running, powerful enkephalins called *endorphins* attach themselves to the receptor sites where normally morphine or other opiates would attach, thus blocking the feeling of pain.

Thus we have the familiar "runner's high"—that great feeling of well-being that a runner experiences at some point during his run, that fills him with a false sense of euphoria. If the body does not produce enough enkephalins and the receptor sites are not filled, then the runner might experience a feeling of irritation or urgency.

When there is an overabundance of this production, we might feel euphoric, then let down. Drugs such as heroin or morphine can take the place of these endorphins and enkephalins at the receptor sites. These drugs block the receptor sites for long periods of time because they don't get broken down and recycled like the natural opiates produced by the body.

So we feel "high," or we just enjoy a sense of well-being. Now, here's the rub. When someone uses heroin or morphine, there is no need for the body to manufacture endorphins or enkephalins and no place to store them at the receptor sites, even if they were being made. When the drugs (heroin, morphine) wear off, the feeling of need is greater than ever, and drug dependence is formed.

Now enter the villain, THIQ! This is the code name for a chemical called tetrahydroisoquiniline (now you know why we just refer to it as THIQ) that is formed by alcohol along with other chemicals called alkaloids; they all have the same effect as morphine and heroin. THIQ is manufactured during the consumption of alcohol, attaching itself to and filling the receptor sites. The body's production of endorphins and enkephalins is thereby reduced, and alcohol addiction occurs.

The THIQ and the alkaloids thus produced are thought to be "super addicting." Once the THIQs are formed as a result of drinking alcohol, they remain in the body. Even after years of abstinence, once alcohol is consumed again, the THIQs reactivate, causing the alcoholic to drink compulsively.

One of the apparent genetic differences between

alcoholics and non-alcoholics seems to be in brain chemistry. Alcoholics produce fewer endorphins and enkephalins to start with, and, of course, the production of these substances is further reduced by the presence of alcohol, hence the addicting effect of THIQ. But that's not all. Stress is a big factor in this curtailed production, and that alters body chemistry even more. Stress might be the trigger that leads to alcohol consumption. So a vicious circle develops: chronic stress occurs, triggering the drinking of alcohol, which promotes the changes in the chemicals in the brain, causing more stress, leading to more alcohol abuse.

Well, naturally, biochemists have been hard at work seeking new methods to correct this endorphin and enkephalin deficiency, in the hopes of eliminating the craving for the alcohol. Of course, there are some real hazards: the endorphins and enkephalins cannot be administered in pill form because they are really proteins. Digestive enzymes would attack them, breaking them down into amino acids, just as they do meat.

Prescription drugs can be taken to encourage the body to produce more endorphins and enkephalins, but these drugs are themselves highly addicting. One of the other approaches being used is to load the body with amino acids, the substances from which endorphins and enkephalins are made.

The idea here is to stimulate the body's production of endorphins and enkephalins, load up the receptor sites, and thus reduce the craving for alcohol. This is a very new theory that has yet to be tested. However, an eager pharmaceutical company already has a product on the market that claims to do the trick.

The product itself consists of four amino acids and some vitamins. It supposedly blocks the enzymes that break down the endorphins and enkephalins. Further, this product is supposed to encourage the formation of extra amounts of these chemicals. Unfortunately, the theory behind the product is still unproved.

We'll continue to say it: There is no known cure for alcoholism, and certainly none that is contained in one pill or one method of treatment. Alcoholism is a multi-faceted disease requiring a holistic treatment, embracing physical, psychological, spiritual, environmental, genetic, and certainly emotional aspects of life.

THE HYPOGLYCEMIC DIET THEORY

"Hypoglycemia" is a big word for low blood sugar. One theory that has been advanced suggests that alcoholics are hypoglycemic and should therefore follow a special diet.

There's no evidence to support the fact that all or even most alcoholics are hypoglycemic, but let's look at some facts behind this theory. As we've told you, the use of alcohol causes fluctuations in the level of sugar in the blood. When a person drinks, the blood sugar level rises and then drops in a manner resembling hypoglycemia.

When blood sugar (glucose) levels rise, as they do after eating and particularly after sweets are consumed, the pancreas secretes insulin to bring these levels down. The insulin also causes the extra sugar to be converted into body starch (glycogen). Glycogen is then stored in the liver and muscles of our body until it is needed.

In this process, energy is not lost; glucose is stored for periods of fasting, such as at night. If the body starch reserves start to get low, then body protein and fat are converted into glucose, enabling the brain to continue functioning. When these chemical events occur, there is energy for normal activities.

Now here comes our drinker. He or she is consuming alcohol to excess. Meals are being skipped or they are being eaten on an irregular basis. Because alcohol contains large amounts of sugar, blood sugar levels fluctuate; the alcohol raises the level temporarily, remember, and then drops it to levels below "normal."

When alcohol is in the body, body starch (glycogen) is not formed, enzymes from the pancreas are unable to function, and you start getting into trouble. Because the glycogen cannot be formed in the presence of alcohol, there are no "reserve troops" available for being converted into glucose for quick energy. If the alcoholic is not drinking, he or she needs this energy.

If low blood sugar reactions present themselves, the alcoholic is frequently unaware of them and just continues to drink more in order to avoid feeling faint, dizzy, or unable to cope.

Body organs and enzymes do not just shape up immediately once the drinking person decides to enter sobriety. A rather slow "pony express" carries the message around the body, informing each of the millions and millions of cells that they now have to learn to function without the alcohol they have grown accustomed to.

Until that message gets around, the body is in a kind of quandary—it doesn't know exactly what to do and fluctuates from one extreme to another. Blood sugar levels jump from high to low without warning. In the early stages of recovery, we see patients stuffing themselves with massive doses of sugar.

Sweets become the order of the day. Once you may have drunk your coffee hot and black; now it becomes a syrupy mess loaded with sugar. Ice cream, pop, and candy become high-priority items, and people who rarely had desserts before now crave them as much as, or more than, the main meal itself.

What we are seeing here is simply the body's struggle to keep the blood sugar (glucose) levels up so it can function. The problem is that what starts out as self-preservation can quickly turn into an addiction. In an ideal world, the many regulatory centers of the body would get the message that there is life without alcohol, and that they need to start figuring out a way to maintain those blood sugar levels without the booze immediately. As it is, changes in these regulatory centers begin being felt only after the first two to six weeks of sobriety. The panic of having to meet sugar needs without alcohol subsides, and less sugary foods begin to fulfill the body's need for glucose.

Would you believe that foods such as breads, potatoes, pasta, tomatoes, broccoli, in addition to fruit and fruit juices can satisfy your "sugary" needs? Well, they can. If you are following the hypoglycemic diet, no concentrated sugar is allowed. Meals are smaller and eaten more frequently.

We instruct all our patients to try six small meals a day, instead of three big ones, thus helping regulate the large doses of sugar that we dump into our systems. This hypoglycemic regime does seem to help some recovering persons regain their stability more easily. Caution! We are certainly not suggesting that all alcoholics are hypoglycemic and should therefore follow this diet. A recovering person can eat small amounts more frequently as a means of helping to maintain blood sugar levels.

THE ALLERGY THEORY

This theory was proposed a number of years ago, but not much happened with it until recently. It's a pretty simple theory, actually. It has to do with the fact that alcohol is made from, and mixed with, foods. Corn, wheat, potatoes, grapes, and berries are mixed with yeast to produce alcoholic beverages. If you combine alcohol with other foods such as peaches, citrus juices, and tomatoes, for example, you are combining it with foods that have the potential to cause allergic reactions.

A physician, Theron Randolph, wrote in 1979 about food fractions found in alcohol that are rapidly absorbed from the stomach and intestine due to the presence of the alcohol, which, you will recall, requires no digestion. Dr. Randolph theorized that alcoholism or the craving for alcohol, might actually be a craving for the substance from which it was made or with which it was mixed. Therefore, Dr. Randolph advanced the idea that if a recovering person abstained from the substance or substances from which his alcoholic drink was made, as well as from the alcohol itself, the craving for alcohol would disappear.

His proposed method of treatment involves eliminating the foods to which one is allergic, as well as those from which the common alcoholic beverages are made. We strongly suggest that in following this regimen you rotate all the food groups, so that allergic responses to other foods will be less likely to develop.

Of course, as in other "magical" methods, a lot of alcoholics reason that if they simply avoid drinking the beverages that contain foods to which they might be allergic, they can go on merrily drinking alcoholic beverages from other food groups and not drink compulsively. The mind of the alcoholic is, to say the least, diabolically clever even though misled.

We do have reports that seem to support Randolph's theory, possibly because the general level of stress is reduced when certain foods to which you may be allergic are eliminated. You certainly feel better when you leave the stable during hay fever season, if you are allergic to hay. In like manner, just reducing the stress load will help the alcoholic maintain sobriety.

THE YEAST SYNDROME THEORY

This theory is closely allied to the one just detailed. It is based on the belief that using substances, such as alcohol, that disrupt the body's immune system and cause an imbalance between the yeast and the bacterial colonies of the intestines, promotes a sensitivity to yeasts and molds.

Get the picture? Alcoholic beverages are fermented and are produced by adding yeast or a culture to foods.

Taking this theory to its limit, any food or beverage that is high in yeast or mold will creat a craving for alcohol. It does this by causing a type of allergic reaction.

It is known that some persons who are allergic to yeast and mold are alcoholic, have an alcoholic family history, and do not tolerate alcohol. The beer drinker, consuming can after can of a beverage that is high in yeast, may also be found to be very sensitive to yeast and mold.

Some persons find that eliminating foods that are high in yeast and mold from their diets helps their sobriety along. They will banish from their tables cheese, vinegar and any foods containing it, breads such as sourdough, buttermilk, yogurt, soy sauce, sauerkraut, and prepared foods that have been made from moldy or very ripe fruits.

Obviously, for devotees of this theory, yeast extract and yeast flavorings are also off limits. Many recovering people find this diet rather limited, more limited than they can handle, and they may avoid using it even if it seems to help. However, it is not harmful and might just fit into your lifestyle.

THE NATURAL-FOODS DIET THEORY

Here's the last of the various theories about nutrition and alcoholism. In its most liberal form, the natural-foods diet includes liberal amounts of fruits and vegetables, some of which are to be eaten raw every day.

Some advocates of this diet believe that everything must be eaten raw or grown without chemical fertilizers. Others will abstain from meat, poultry, eggs, fish, and milk, while other disciples of this diet make their variations on this theme, making sure that their meats are low in fat.

The grains used in this diet are whole grains, not refined ones. Food is processed just enough to make it taste good. Convenience foods are avoided (except for special or unusual occasions).

People using this diet wait for the holidays to even think about fried foods, gravies, sauces, and similar items. Sugar and foods containing sugar are not eaten daily. Some go so far as to avoid all foods in which sugar is among the first five ingredients listed.

Recognize this diet? It's very similar to the one recommended for reducing your chances of heart disease. It's also similar to the cancer-fighting diet and the one recommended in the U.S. Dietary Guidelines. The key to this, or any other program used in your recovery, is to make gradual changes so you can take care of your physical needs during the recovery process.

Nutritional supplements may or may not be included as part of this diet, but you may find some advocates of the natural-foods diet "thumping the tub" for megadoses of vitamins and minerals. However, anything more than three times the Recommended Daily Allowance (RDA) is wasted and in some instances can alter your body chemistry so that you become dependent upon these megadoses.

When you are taking five to ten times the RDA, some nutrients act as drugs rather than as nutrients. Some persons have experienced deficiency symptoms as a consequence of taking megadoses and then eliminating them. Generally speaking, a one-a-day vitamin-mineral supplement is safe, as well as low-potency B complex, vitamin C, and minerals.

One other aspect of the natural-foods diet involves the use of herbs. The idea here is that since herbs are "natural," they can't do any harm. The fact is that many of our modern medications originally come from herbs, so they can be toxic.

No, you don't have to avoid the herb teas found in your supermarket, unless, of course, you are allergic to them. However, when you take herbs found in health-food stores in bulk or in pill form for medicinal purposes, you need to be aware of the possible side effects.

One of the herbs frequently recommended (strangely enough) for recovering persons is valarian. It is dangerous and potentially addicting, as are a few other herbs.

The recovering person should *always* consult a treatment professional in these matters. As we said at the beginning of this chapter, there are a lot of "snake oil" salesmen out there and they represent a clear and present danger to your program of recovery.

Whew! We've laid some pretty heavy material on you in this chapter, material we hope will help clarify some of the things you may have heard or read about as treatments for alcoholism. Just keep in mind that you are constantly treating a disease and that this disease has no known cure. We want you to understand some of the theories concerning the relationship of nutrition to a successful recovery from alcoholism.

3
Decisions! Decisions!
What Do I Eat?

As a recovering person, you may be finding that you are giving consideration to taking care of yourself for a change. In contrast to the self-destructive patterns of your drinking, you now need to reexamine your eating habits and learn to choose the good foods that will promote lifelong sobriety.

That's what this chapter is all about: helping you learn about basic foods so you can make the right choices at the grocery store. So let's start with some review of things you probably learned in school and then promptly forgot.

There are four basic food groups: fruits and vegetables; grains; dairy foods; and meat, fish, poultry, and eggs. Each of us needs to have foods from each of these groups on a daily basis in order to ensure that our bodies will obtain sufficient amounts of nutrients.

Because alcoholism has caused some drastic physical changes in the body, you will need to pay closer attention to certain food groups than to others, as well as taking a closer look at the amounts of the foods consumed. So let's begin with some discussion of the food group that is most often neglected by Americans in general and by alcoholics in particular. This is the fruits and vegetables category.

FRUITS AND VEGETABLES

The recommended number of servings from this group for the average person is from four to six a day. If you are recovering, then we suggest you lean toward the higher figure. Why? Because fruits and vegetables are our primary source of vitamins A and C and of fiber. As we have previously discussed, the alcohol that has been consumed has either interfered with or washed away these two important vitamins. Fruits and vegetables will help restore these lost vitamins.

At least one daily serving from this group needs to be high in a yellow coloring matter called carotene. Our bodies convert carotene into vitamin A and also use the carotene itself to strengthen the mucous membrane lining the mouth, esophagus, stomach, intestines, trachea, and lungs.

Recent research shows that carotene offers some protection against cancer, especially lung cancer. You should have at least one reasonably large serving of high-carotene foods daily. Now, how do you know which fruits and vegetables contain this carotene? Well, look at the color. The darker the color of the fruit or vegetable, the more carotene it contains. Why? Because the longer the food item is exposed to the sun during the growing process, the greater the amount of carotene it forms. As in everything else, there are exceptions to this rule. Such root vegetables as carrots, beets, and sweet potatoes are all high in carotene but of course are grown below ground. The leaves of these vegetables take in the sun's energy, produce carotene, and then store it in the roots. Think of yourself as an amateur color designer when selecting foods. You can be easily fooled by appearances, though. For example, the yellow color of the carotene is masked by the predominant color of the fruit or vegetable: the reds of tomatoes or beets, the greens of broccoli, spinach, leaf lettuce, and chard.

These vegetables are all good sources of carotene, as are the carrots, sweet potatoes, and winter squash that look yellow and contain carotene. In the fruit department, select peaches, apricots, oranges, cantaloupes, and papaya. Wait! Don't pass up those wonderful red or purple plums. They're high in carotene, too.

How you cook these foods is important, too. You won't destroy the carotene or vitamin A unless you overcook. That's why steaming your vegetables is such a nutritious way to prepare vegetables. The cooking process works to your advantage in such vegetables as carrots, beets, broccoli, and green beans, because as the cellulose in these foods is softened, they become more digestible. This allows your body to absorb more of the carotene than if the foods were eaten raw. Carotene is readily available in raw fruits as well as cooked ones, and the cellulose in fruits is softer than that of vegetables. Carotene in carrot juice is even more available, but here we must sound a note of caution. Too much carrot juice might be toxic if it is consumed daily. In fact, carotene and/or vitamin A in large amounts interfere with the absorption of other nutrients. This is a good time to mention serving sizes. If your fruit or vegetable is raw, plan on 1 cup per serving and ½ to ¾ cup, if cooked.

Vitamin C is more easily destroyed or altered so that the body cannot use it. Therefore, we want to emphasize those fruits and vegetables that have higher concentrations of this vitamin. Raw fruits and vegetables, or those with a minimum amount of processing, are high in vitamin C. We all know that citrus fruits are good sources of vitamin C. Have you considered or do you even know about these sources: tomatoes, cabbage, cauliflower, broccoli, brussels sprouts, and raw green pepper? One-quarter of a raw green pepper provides the essential daily requirement of vitamin C. Keep it in mind the next time you shop.

Some other foods high in vitamin C might also surprise you. Baked white potato, strawberries, cantaloupe, and other summer fruits in season yield vitamin C. Vitamin C, you'll remember, is water soluble. It is also altered by heat and air, which means fruits and vegetables should not be soaked in water for long periods of time.

If they are cooked, use minimum amounts of water and only enough cooking time to soften the vegetable slightly. Try for that nice plate of crisp vegetables instead of the mushy ones. Now, this may upset you a lot if you're a mashed potato lover, but you should realize that when you whip up those potatoes, you are whipping air into them and therefore losing almost all the vitamin C. The same loss occurs when you shred that head of cabbage for your favorite coleslaw. If you must cut up fruits and vegetables, learn to cut into larger pieces to help preserve the vitamin C. The larger the piece, the more vitamin C is conserved, because less surface is exposed to air and water.

You may want to change the way you have been mixing up those frozen concentrated orange juices. You know, mixing in enough water to make a big pitcher. Try mixing just enough for what you will consume immediately, because storing the full pitcher in your refrigerator will cause some loss of vitamin C.

How much vitamin C do you need? One to two servings a day of raw fruit (the ones high in vitamin C) are recommended. If you are a recovering person, make it two. If you smoke, then increase the number of servings from two to three, since smoking inhibits the body's ability to store vitamin C, among other things.

Serving sizes should be ½ to 1 cup of juice and ¾ to 1 cup of fruit or vegetable.

When we eat at least one fruit or vegetable high in carotene, and several raw fruits and vegetables to pick up our vitamin C, then we can look to other fruits and vegetables for the so-called trace minerals such as potassium. Potassium is one of those minerals that the alcoholic frequently lacks. Bananas are a good source of this mineral.

WHOLE GRAINS

This group of foods is the major source of B-complex vitamins, as well as being a good source of zinc, magnesium, and selenium. Whole grains are rich in dietary fiber, a nutrient essential to the healthful elimination of body wastes.

The recovering alcoholic especially needs this group of foods since his or her drinking has pretty much depleted body stores of most of the B-complex vitamins. Daily intake should be from three to four servings from this food group, following these serving sizes: ½ cup cooked grain, ¾ cup prepared or cold cereal, and one slice of bread. You may adjust upward, of course, for your appetite or caloric needs.

What we want to emphasize is the whole grain rather than the refined one. When the bran is removed in the course of making white flour or refined cereals such as Cream of Wheat, the process also removes 90 percent of the vitamins and minerals, as well as the fiber. So it becomes necessary to replace the missing vitamins B_1, B_2, niacin, and even perhaps iron and calcium. However, the fiber and other nutrients are not replaced.

You really have to turn into a detective when shopping for breads in your local store. Breads whose labels tell you that they "contain more fiber than whole-wheat bread," contain nonfood cellulose, and the cellulose used is obtained from wood pulp, not from grain. True enough, the weight in fiber is there, and there is more fiber than the grain originally contained, but the fiber used interferes with the body's absorption of calcium, magnesium, and zinc—vital ingredients for the recovering person.

Ready for more sleuthing? "Wheat bread" does not mean whole-wheat bread; it means that the bread is made from wheat flour, which can be either white or whole wheat. So what do you do when you want whole wheat? Read the list of ingredients for your set of clues. The law requires that ingredients be listed in descending order of weight. So look for the first ingredient to be whole-wheat flour.

If, under your magnifying glass, you read first "wheat flour" or "unbleached flour," then "whole-wheat flour," you are about to put a loaf of essentially white bread (with enough whole-wheat flour to provide a chewy texture) into your shopping cart.

"Aha, Watson!" you cry, "the game is afoot!" You go on to note, "These breads are dark in color, they even look as if they are whole grain!"

"How so, Holmes?" remarks a perplexed Watson. "How can they be dark in color if they are not whole wheat?"

"Elementary, my dear Watson. Caramel coloring has been added, as you can plainly read on the list of ingredients.

"Whole-grain rye bread is what we are after, Watson," you continue, now well into your detective work. "But this rye bread is really white bread with just enough rye flour added to give us some rye flavor, with perhaps a bit of caramel coloring."

Whole-grain rye bread is very heavy and doesn't fit the average American's concept of bread. So we find a good deal of the rye bread being sold in supermarkets to be essentially white bread with rye flavoring, to cater to American tastes.

Use the same rules for choosing your cereals as you use for choosing your bread. That first ingredient should be a whole grain (in some instances it will be the only ingredient). Be aware of the sugar content of most cold cereals and of a few cereals intended for cooking. It isn't unusual to find prepared cereals that contain 40 to 60 percent sugar or sweeteners of some other type. Chapter 11 will deal in greater detail with sugar.

You'll save time in your shopping once you begin to read labels. By limiting your selections to whole-grain products with little or no sugar, you narrow down the range of possible purchases. You'll also discover that the cost will be a little higher with the whole grains, but you get a bonus in greater appetite satisfaction. The high-fiber content of whole-grain breads and cereals lets you eat less, but enjoy more. Makes sense, doesn't it? Next time you are hankering to lose some weight (who isn't?) or adjust what you have, you will find whole grains to be an important part of your diet. You won't feel as hungry when you eat these foods.

While we are talking about whole grains, let's go into the starches that we use as "side dishes." We suggest you use brown rice instead of white. Whole-grain pasta should be on your table. However, be warned! If you were to be sitting with the hungry brood at the Hatcher house, you might hear plenty of booing for whole-wheat pasta. Why this reaction? Because if it is not cooked and served immediately, whole-wheat pasta becomes mushy. One exception: whole-wheat lasagna noodles. Most of us don't have schedules that allow for such accurate timing, so white-flour pasta frequently becomes the first choice.

Brown rice is something else, however. It takes about 45 minutes to cook; it is chewy as compared to the smooth texture of white rice. You can cook it in the oven, which saves the watching you have to do with white rice. If it should cook dry, brown rice just toasts and resembles fried rice, thus making it no less acceptable as a "side dish." If you burn rice, you have to throw it away, vowing to find a way to watch it closer next time.

When you substitute whole-grain flour for white flour in a recipe, you also change the flavor and the texture of the final product. You can experiment and get interesting and tasty results. Whole-grain flour is drier than white, so you should use slightly less of it or add slightly more liquid.

DAIRY FOODS

The dairy foods group is important to us because of our need for calcium. Milk and foods made from milk are our best sources of calcium. Calcium, which makes strong bones and teeth, is of particular concern to the recovering female. The alcohol disrupts calcium absorption, which in turn may affect bone loss. Men generally do not have bone loss until after the age of 50.

Adult men up to the age of 35 should be consuming 800 milligrams of calcium a day. Women require 1,000 milligrams a day until the start of menopause, when their daily requirement can jump to 1,500 depending on their estrogen levels. Estrogen increases the body's ability to deposit calcium in bones. As your estrogen levels fluctuate with pregnancy and menstruation, so will your calcium requirements change.

A serving of dairy food should consist of 8 ounces of milk or yogurt or 1½ to 2 ounces of cheese. With this serving, you are getting approximately 300 milligrams of calcium. At this rate, two or three servings of dairy products per day will supply you with your basic calcium needs. If you're going for "peak intake" of calcium, to meet the higher requirement strictly from food, you will have to raise the number of servings of dairy foods to five per day.

Ice cream is not a dairy food. It is 50 percent air and high in sugar, fat, and calories. When you add up all these negatives about ice cream, you realize it isn't a very good source of calcium. We acknowledge that it does quite a bit to satisfy our bodies' needs for "rewards," though.

Skim milk, lower in saturated fat and calories, is often preferred as a source of calcium. Skim milk is also fortified with vitamin A to replace what is lost when the cream is removed. Milk and cheese are used freely in cooking, in addition to being eaten plain. Some folks use extra powdered milk in muffins or biscuits, and pour melted cheeses generously over hot vegetable dishes.

The calcium you get from dairy foods may be a problem for you as a recovering person. You may have a lactose-tolerance problem, but you can use cheese and yogurt instead of milk. Milk that has been treated with an enzyme to digest the lactose is also available in many supermarkets. So you can still have milk on your morning cereal.

If, however, you can't tolerate milk in any form, or if you can't eat the recommended amount of calcium without gaining weight, then a calcium supplement is in order. Calcium carbonate is the calcium supplement most often recommended, because it is 40 percent calcium. Stay away from Tums or other antacids as sources of calcium because the same substances in these products that are used to combat excessive acid also interfere with calcium absorption.

MEAT, FISH, POULTRY, AND EGGS

Meat, fish, poultry, and eggs, along with milk and cheese, provide complete proteins that are essential for the body's maintenance. Would you be surprised to learn that your daily protein needs can be met with 4 to 6 (or at the most 8) ounces of these foods? Well, they can! Of course, when you eat out, most restaurants will serve 4 to 12 ounces of these foods, so we become trained to want larger servings than we actually need, at least as far as meeting minimum daily requirements is concerned.

While these foods provide protein, they are also high in fat and therefore high in calories. Even when all the visible fat has been trimmed, 20 to 30 percent of calories are found in the fat distributed between meat fibers. If you are into fish, white fish has less fat than darker fish. Since the foods in this group are by far the most expensive items in our shopping carts, we probably can afford to use less of them. We can substitute high-carbohydrate foods such as fruits, vegetables, and grains.

We have all been exposed to campaigns urging us to use less red meat and more fish and poultry. The fat in beef, lamb, and pork is saturated. When we have a high intake of saturated fats, we are encouraging our bodies to make cholesterol, thus increasing the risk of coronary heart disease.

There is a general perception of eggs as a high-cholesterol food. For persons who are concerned about their cholesterol, three eggs per week (or fewer) seem in order. One egg is the equivalent of 1 ounce of meat, as far as calories and protein are concerned. If cholesterol is not a problem for you, then eggs are a valuable and relatively inexpensive source of protein. While we are talking about fat, the fat on poultry is less saturated and is not distributed between lean meat fibers as the fat in red meat is. You can remove the fat more easily, and keeping fat out of your diet is very important for self-care and for reducing the risk of heart disease.

If you can manage to eat salmon, mackerel, cod, or herring once or twice a week, you will be eating fat that reduces cholesterol. A small amount of fat added to foods in the form of butter or salad dressing enhances flavor and makes food more interesting. For most of us, 1 to 2 tablespoons of this fat or oil per day is sufficient.

Sources of Protein for Vegetarians

Many of our ethnic foods, at least the ones found in American diets, are vegetarian. We call a diet vegetarian when two or more vegetable proteins are combined to obtain the same amino acids that are found in fish, poultry, and meat. For example, bean burritos, tacos, red beans and rice, pinto beans and corn bread, bolitos, posole, and macaroni and cheese are some favorites that come to mind.

If a vegetarian diet contains no dairy foods and no meat, fish, or poultry, then supplements might be called for. However, if some animal foods are included and the emphasis is on vegetarian protein foods, then you'll get a lower-fat/higher-fiber intake. All of this would naturally lead to improved health.

KEEPING THE BAD GUYS IN CHECK
Cholesterol, Triglycerides, and Lipoproteins

Two elements of concern for everyone, but especially for you as a recovering person, are cholesterol and triglycerides. It's likely that when you were examined during your active drinking stage, your doctor or clinician used your levels of cholesterol and triglycerides to assess your physical condition. So let's look at these two elements in a little greater detail.

Cholesterol is a fatty substance produced by the body, primarily in the liver. It's also provided by some foods. Cholesterol is not entirely bad; it performs a number of essential functions. And the body produces a number of essential substances from cholesterol. For example, bile, the substance that we use for the digestion of fats, is a product of cholesterol. Steroids, including corticoids, which prevent inflammation, are products of cholesterol. So are sex hormones and vitamin D.

So you see, there is some good in cholesterol.

High blood levels of cholesterol, however, tend to form deposits in your blood vessels and therefore restrict the area available for blood flow. Result? Your blood pressure goes up. This increase in pressure, plus the cholesterol deposits, causes hardening of the arteries.

Taking this a step or two further, let's suppose that a cholesterol deposit enlarges, restricting blood flow even more. Suppose a blood clot catches on one of these cholesterol deposits, then what? Well, if that happens, blood supply is drastically reduced or cut off entirely, possibly resulting in severe damage to vital organs.

Loss of blood to your heart is what we mean by a "heart attack." If the blood supply to the brain is severely restricted, then we say someone is having a "stroke." High cholesterol levels have been directly linked to heart attacks and strokes. When you take into account the fairly sedentary American lifestyle and the high fat content of the average diet, you can see that cholesterol poses a serious problem. The average American, who obtains 42 percent of his total calories from high-fat foods, has high blood cholesterol levels.

Cholesterol is manufactured in your body primarily from saturated fats, the ones that stay solid at room temperature. The main sources of cholesterol are egg yolk, liver and other organ meats, butter, and shellfish. Saturated fats are found primarily in red meat, butter, cream, and coconut and palm kernel oils.

So we have seen a great trend toward the use of polyunsaturated fats in our daily diets. These are the *good* fats—the kind that lower cholesterol levels. These substances are primarily vegetable oils that are liquid at room temperature. Olive and peanut oil are monounsaturated fats and do not affect cholesterol levels. When you are grocery shopping keep in mind that the oils highest in polyunsaturated fats are safflower, sunflower, corn, and soy.

When you see "vegetable oil" listed as one of the ingredients in a product you may be buying, it doesn't mean that one of these oils was used. In fact, coconut and palm kernel oil are frequently cheaper and less likely to turn rancid, so producers, especially bakeries, tend to use these saturated vegetable oils more than unsaturated ones.

Purchase oils that tell you specifically that they are not those just labeled vegetable oil. However, when vegetable oils are solidified (hydrogenated) to make shortening and margarine, they act like saturated fats and become as detrimental to your health as beef tallow or lard. You will find some squeeze or tub margarines to be partially hydrogenated.

Triglycerides also increase the risk of heart disease. Your body's supply of these comes primarily from high-fat foods, high alcohol consumption, and foods high in sugar. When triglyceride levels are within normal limits there is no health concern. Elevated triglyceride levels alone do not indicate the risk of heart disease. However, when you find other conditions such as obesity, diabetes, smoking, high blood pressure, high cholesterol levels, and/or a family history of heart disease, your triglyceride levels become a cause for concern.

So what are triglycerides, anyway? Well, triglycerides, which make up the major part of body fat, are composed of glycerol, which is an alcohol, and three fatty acids, thus *tri*glyceride. All glyceride molecules are the same, but the fatty acids may vary in length or degree of saturation. Triglycerides are used for energy—you need them! They are also the form in which body fat is stored. When the levels of triglycerides are higher, there is also higher risk of heart disease.

You can lower your triglyceride levels in several ways. You can lose weight, if you are obese. You can decrease the amount of fat you eat, while increasing your fiber intake. You can participate in some form of aerobic exercise three to five times a week. You can stop smoking. Needless to say, you should consult your physician and follow his or her advice when attempting to lower your triglyceride levels.

Lipoproteins are compounds of protein and fat that the body forms so that fat can be transported by the blood. One of the new tools being used in diagnostic medicine is the "coronary risk profile," which measures, in addition to your cholesterol and triglycerides, two kinds of lipoproteins: HDL (high-density lipoproteins) and LDL (low-density lipoproteins). The good lipoproteins are the HDL, high-density lipoproteins, because they are low in fat and high in proteins. LDL and another one called VLDL, which stands for very low density lipoproteins, are the culprits. They are higher in fat and pose a greater risk for coronary heart disease.

You will probably use the same methods to increase HDL and lower LDL or VLDL that we described for lowering your triglycerides. What can you do at home? Well, cut away all visible fat from meat before you cook. Don't deep-fry or use large amounts of fats or oils in cooking. Instead, get in the habit of baking, broiling, or stewing meat. Treat breaded and fried foods, or those with sauces other than tomato, as special holiday fare treats. Avoid them in your daily diet.

Fat

If we are to really toe the line of nutritional health, we should consume very little fat. Putting this into concrete terms, we should avoid gravies and sauces (except tomato sauce) and use minimal amounts of salad dressings and butter for seasoning or as a spread for bread. Needless to say, fried foods are a real no-no.

Salt

Salt is another nutritional troublemaker. The average intake is three times what is needed for good health.

Prepared foods are the primary sources of salt. For example, just half a can of soup contains more than half the daily requirement of salt. If we added no salt to our foods and used bread and butter or margarine that contain salt, we would meet all our salt needs for one day. Don't start being a "great reformer" on salt; decrease the amount you use gradually and give your taste buds a chance to adjust.

Ham, bacon, lunch meat, pickles, olives, chips, and crackers are all pretty heavy in the salt department. Ideally, we should use these foods only occasionally.

Sugar

Sugar is a term used to describe sucrose, cane sugar, or beet sugar. It occurs naturally in many foods that we eat, including fruits, vegetables, and, of course, maple syrup, molasses, and sorghum. White sugar has been refined to remove impurities and color. Brown sugar originally was less refined white sugar, but today it is white sugar with molasses added to give it its color and flavor.

Molasses is really sugar syrup that is less refined than sugar. It contains minerals and may or may not be bleached. It is in the syrup section in supermarkets. Raw sugar is partially refined sugar that contains a lot of molasses or sucrose that has not yet been bleached. For all practical purposes, it is refined white sugar. You may also find this product under the name of "turbinado" sugar. It is not always available in supermarkets and its cost is exorbitant.

Honey is also a simple sugar. Honey contains small amounts of vitamins and minerals, but not really enough to add significant amounts to the diet. It tastes sweeter than sugar and you should therefore use less of it, even though most people substitute it in equal amounts for sugar, therefore getting as much sweetener as they did from other sources, or more.

Now, at first glance, you might think that the concentrated fruit juices (containing fructose), which are presently being used to sweeten some baked goods, are better than sugar. But when you realize that fructose is sugar, whether it comes in the form of fruit or a refined powder, then the idea of using it in large amounts makes less sense. Fructose in fruit concentrate is essentially a refined sugar.

Fructose tastes sweeter than sucrose, so less of it can be used to give the same amount of sweetness. Fructose in nature is found in fruits and is therefore thought of as a "natural" sweetener. But in its refined form, it is no different that sucrose. About five years ago, a process for producing fructose economically was introduced and perfected. For a short time, it was thought that persons who were diabetic or hypoglycemic might be able to use fructose, because insulin is not secreted when fructose is present. However, when it was found that fructose is converted by the body into glucose (blood sugar), which triggers the release of insulin, fructose turned out to be no more beneficial than any of the other forms of sugar.

The American public is greatly concerned about sugar and the very possible negative impact of its overuse on overall health. The food industry has responded by de-emphasizing the amount of sugar present in foods, and by using many different terms to describe sugar. As a smart shopper, you know that ingredients are listed in descending order of weight on food packages. Here comes the "sugar bind." If you are not aware of all the names for sugar, you might not realize that sugar is a major ingredient if it is not among the first listed. But beware! Other types of sugar might appear at the beginning of the ingredients list. What other types?

Generally, words ending with *ose* indicate a form of sugar. Thus, processed foods might list levul*ose*, fruct*ose*, dextr*ose*, lact*ose*, malt*ose*, as well as corn syrup, invert sugar, corn sweetener, honey, molasses, malt syrup, sorghum, and sugar itself. More work for Holmes and Watson, eh?

An ingredient containing sugar might have been added but its sugar content not noted. "Sugar-free" or "sugarless" might mean that no sucrose has been used, although the food you are selecting might very well contain glucose, corn syrup, fructose, or any number of other sugars.

Well, you can see why we keep stressing that the foods you prepare at home are more under your control than anything you pick up at the stores or in restaurants. Here are some other foods that contain sugar:

Stuffing and bread mixes
Canned and dried soups
Peanut butter
Frozen pizza
Soy sauce
Gravy mixes
Dips for chips
Salad dressings
Meat tenderizers
Spices
Frozen and canned vegetables
Frozen dinners
Bouillon cubes
Garlic salt
Cereals
Crackers
Table salt

When you eat 8 ounces of yogurt, you get 6 teaspoons of sugar. One ounce of cold cereal contains 2 to 5 teaspoons of sugar, and your favorite soda of 12 ounces contains 10 to 12 teaspoons of sugar. Can you see how easy it is for you to pack away your 120 pounds of sugar per year?

There is no need to feel deprived when these dietary decisions are made. Experimenting with herbs and spices will add new flavor dimensions to your foods. Changing your eating habits must be thought of as a gradual process, not as a goal to be reached immediately. There is no instant cure for these dietary and nutritional problems. Just keep plugging away at the guidelines we have provided for purchasing and using the basic food groups.

Here's a handy summary and a typical day's menu, with some snacks thrown in for good behavior—*your* good behavior!

SUMMARY

Fruits and vegetables: Four to six servings daily. At least one serving should be high in carotene or vitamin A, and two or more servings should be high in vitamin C. At least one and preferably two servings should be raw.

Whole-grain breads and cereals: Three to four servings daily.

Dairy products: Two to five servings daily, depending on calcium needs. Skim milk, low-fat yogurt, or cheese provide about half the calories found in full-fat dairy foods.

Meat, fish, poultry, and eggs: Two to three servings daily. Two-to-four-ounce portions provide enough protein. If dairy is not used, this amount should be increased by 1 ounce per dairy serving suggested. No more than 3 ounces total needs to be added. The emphasis is on lean meat with all visible fat removed. Cook without added fat.

Seasonings: Use herbs and spices instead of salt and pepper. Use fats, oils, salt, and sugar in minimal amounts.

Water: Six to eight glasses (1½ quarts) daily. This does not include coffee, tea, or milk.

MENU SUGGESTIONS

Breakfast
½ cup Shredded Wheat
12 ounces 2 percent milk
Fresh fruit
Slice whole-wheat toast, if desired

Lunch
Sandwich: 2 to 3 ounces turkey, two slices
whole-wheat bread, tomato, lettuce, mustard, and minimal amount of mayonnaise
Fresh fruit
8 ounces 2 percent milk

Dinner
2 to 3 ounces lean roast beef au jus
Baked potato
Steamed broccoli
Tossed salad: leaf lettuce, tomato, cucumber,
green pepper, etc., with minimal amount of
dressing
Whole-wheat roll if desired
Fresh fruit and 4 ounces low-fat yogurt

Snacks
Fresh fruit
Raw sunflower seeds
1 to 2 ounces low-fat cheese, if desired

Note: There is a popular myth that liquids
should not be taken with meals. Unless there is
a medicinal reason, there is no problem with
having two cups of coffee or tea with your
meals or between meals. Water can also be
taken with or between meals.

4
Breaking the Magic Wand: Nutrition Myths and Fancies

"It came like magic in a pint bottle; it was not ecstasy but it was comfort"
—Charles Dickens, *Flora Finching*

Americans tend to be gullible. The great showman P. T. Barnum made a fortune knowing that "there is a sucker born every minute." Schemes abound in our society for everything: "magic cures," potions, legends, myths, "super-sex pills," you name it. Down through the ages, people have sought ways to make things easier through the use of unseen powers, which generally replace hard work and persistence, to reach attainable goals.

The field of nutrition certainly has not escaped this tendency. What we are going to share with you in this chapter are some of the myths—the magic that surrounds food, food supplements, vitamins, and minerals. We've included some that you're undoubtedly familiar with and others that may not have yet crossed your path. Either way, it's good for you, a recovering person,

46

to know that nothing beats hard work in your program of recovery. We know of no magic cure for the disease of alcoholism, and certainly no single pill, vitamin, supplement, or other chemical has been found that can beat your own determination to stay sober. It takes a sound program of physical, spiritual, and nutritional objectives to succeed.

Myth: "The Recommended Daily Allowances are based on the minimum amount needed to prevent deficiency diseases. The amounts recommended are too low for most of us, so supplemental vitamins and minerals are essential to maintain health." Now the grabber that's aimed at you, the recovering person: *"Since alcoholics have damaged their bodies, they need megadoses."*

Fact: The RDA is a set of figures based on the amount of essential nutrients needed to prevent deficiency diseases, plus a safety margin of 50 to 60 percent. True, the alcoholic has damaged his or her body and has depleted some essential nutrients. For this reason there may be a period of time when you will need extra B-complex vitamins, zinc, and magnesium.

However, under normal circumstances, you don't need megadoses of anything. Some of you might even be sensitive to megadoses of some of the fat-soluble vitamins and would definitely have adverse reactions to large doses.

Myth: *"Vitamin supplements from natural sources are better than those from chemical sources and are worth the higher price."*

Fact: Vitamins from food are better than those in capsules and tablets. So-called natural vitamins come from the chemist's lab also. If you will read the labels carefully, you will find a list of vitamins in a base of alfalfa meal, liver powder, bone meal, and brewer's yeast. One company trumpets that their alfalfa is grown, harvested, then ground into powder and combined with vitamins from an unidentified source.

The primary difference between so-called natural vitamins and generic ones is in the binder or binders used. There's no substitute for reading the label carefully to determine exactly what you are buying.

Myth: "Synthetic vitamins can be toxic and therefore must be used carefully or avoided altogether. Those from natural sources will be eliminated if too much is taken, so an overdose is impossible."

Fact: "The source of the vitamins does not determine whether or not toxic doses are possible. It's the amount consumed that makes a dose toxic, and it's just as possible to overdose on vitamins from foods as well as those from tablets.

Myth: "You must take vitamin supplements because our soils are so depleted that the foods grown on them have no vitamins."

Fact: This is a partial truth. Vitamins are made by plants and the amount present in them is determined by the variety of plant, growing conditions, sunlight exposure, temperature, water, and a myriad of other things. In most instances, the plants don't grow as well in depleted soil. However, plants grow well in soil deficient in some things such as iodine, cobalt, and magnesium. If minerals are not present in the soil, they can't be in the plants grown there. If we rely on foods grown only in one place, our diet might be deficient in one or two trace minerals.

Myth: "Vitamin A is good for the eyes and skin. No matter what symptoms you have, vitamin A will take care of it."

Fact: Sorry! Vitamin A will not cure pimples, dry skin, oily skin, or nearsightedness. It is true that vitamin A–deficiency syndromes are noticed in the eyes and skin, principally in night blindness and "shark skin," a condition characterized by excessively dry skin. When it comes to treating acne, a medication called Accutane is used to dry the skin. Accutane is the active form of vitamin A and, in the amount prescribed, is a medication. What you can purchase over the counter does not have the same effect as the medication.

Men and women have searched throughout history for cures to sexual problems. Here are a couple of contemporary myths.

Myth: "*Vitamin E is an aphrodisiac. It prevents sterility in rats, therefore it is the 'sex vitamin.'*"

Fact: It's true that animals deficient in vitamin E are sterile, but there's no proof that this applies to humans. The male alcoholic who is sterile is usually deficient in both vitamin A and/or zinc, both of which are necessary to the formation of sperm.

By the way, vitamin E is said to also slow down the aging process and to protect us against air pollution. So far there is just enough evidence to warrant further investigation of these ideas, but they are not proven facts.

Myth: "*Zinc in megadoses improves your sexual life.*"

Fact: People who are zinc-deficient have little or no interest in sex, but the use of zinc supplements will have no impact on sexual performance unless there is a deficiency. For years you've undoubtedly heard the stories about the magical aphrodisiac powers of oysters. Well, if and when they work, it's because of their high zinc content.

Recovering people may be low in zinc because the alcohol they were using was literally leaching the zinc from their bodies. However, megadoses are certainly not called for, although therapeutic doses might be needed on a temporary basis.

It's interesting to read in the 1985 *Farmer's Almanac* about the XX Rooster Pills advertised to make men "bright-eyed and bushy-tailed." These pills are zinc supplements.

Myth: "*Vitamin D is made in the skin by both humans and cows. Cows don't take baths, so they retain the vitamin D. Taking a bath within 2 hours of being in the sun will wash all the vitamin D away and you will be deficient.*"

Fact: Vitamin D is formed under, not on, the surface

of the skin; therefore it does not wash off. Milk is fortified with vitamin D because it helps the body absorb and use calcium. People who live in sunny climates obtain vitamin D more easily than those who live in colder climates and must therefore drink vitamin D–fortified milk to meet their RDA.

Myth: *"B vitamins in large doses will prevent stress or keep it from affecting your body."*

Fact: As we discussed in the previous chapter on stress, your body will need extra B-complex vitamins, as well as vitamin C and zinc, if you are under physical stress from accident, surgery, burns, etc. There is scientific evidence to support these claims. We do not, however, have any evidence of the need for extra vitamins to carry a person through psychological or emotional stress.

There is mounting evidence that humans use larger amounts of some nutrients when emotional stress continues for a period of time.

Myth: *"Vitamin B_{12} gives you energy."*

Fact: Fatigue is a symptom of B_{12} deficiency, true. But it is also a symptom of a deficiency in iron and other B vitamins. Some people will experience a temporary lift after receiving a shot of Vitamin B_{12}, even if they are not deficient in this vitamin.

If your alcohol abuse has damaged your stomach and made it difficult for you to absorb B_{12}, a B_{12} supplement might be indicated for you. There are accurate blood tests for B_{12} levels, and there is no need to take it if your levels are normal. As in all things, the saying, "If it ain't broke, don't fix it!" applies.

While we're on the subject of B vitamins, another myth that affects the alcoholic particularly is this one:

Myth: *"The use of vitamin B_{15}, pangamic acid, prevents cravings for alcohol and eliminates or reduces shortness of breath."*

Fact: Well, for openers, pangamic acid, or calcium pangamate, is not a vitamin. We get most of these "cure claims" from the U.S.S.R., where the Soviets say that persons who take B$_{15}$ no longer crave booze, and that their athletes who take it have more endurance. So far, none of these claims have been proven.

Myth: *"You cannot overdose on water-soluble nutrients."*

Fact: Taking large doses of anything is not a good idea. Some trace minerals can be toxic if taken in megadoses. You will experience a metallic taste if, indeed, you are overdosing. Water-soluble nutrients such as vitamin C, the B vitamins, and all minerals are not stored in large amounts in your body. Extra amounts are eliminated through the kidneys. So, if you take megadoses for a period of time, your body develops a method of getting rid of the excess, but your body becomes dependent on them. When the dose is suddenly reduced, you go into withdrawal symptoms. You may be depressed or just "not feel well."

A friend once said, "Taking cold remedies helps me get rid of my cold in a week. Taking nothing usually requires about seven days!" Well, with that in mind look at this:

Myth: *"Zinc will cure colds."*

Fact: If you are deficient in zinc, you will have more frequent infections and your wounds will tend to heal more slowly. If you are deficient in zinc, your immune system does not function as well as normal. Zinc might be used to help improve the immune reaction of a person who is very ill. For example, it is used success-fully in treating persons with immune-deficiency diseases such as leukemia.

Even though it improves the immune reaction of a person who is very ill, it will not necessarily help the average person prevent or cure a cold.

Myth: *"There are special tests that will show what nutrients you are deficient in. Therefore, you have to buy supplements."*

Fact: If someone suggests that you take a special new

test to determine your nutritional status, question the scientific validity of such a test. There are a few blood tests for vitamin levels that are accurate. Iron, sodium, and potassium levels in the blood are good indicators of a person's nutritional status. You can get blood tests for vitamins A, D, and E that are accurate, but they are also very expensive. Urine tests for vitamins are usually only done at medical labs and research centers.

Good clinicians who know what questions to ask and what your symptoms mean can usually determine if there are any nutritional deficiencies.

Myth: *"Adults do not need milk. Man is the only being on earth who continues to drink milk after being weaned. It is harmful for adults to drink milk."*

Fact: As we stated earlier, there are some adults who cannot or should not drink milk. However, milk and foods made from it are the primary and most concentrated sources of calcium. This calcium is well absorbed and utilized by the persons who can use it, but since there is a regular turnover of calcium in the body, and calcium in bones does not stay around forever, then food or supplement sources are essential for adults as well as children. Go ahead and drink milk.

But now from the sublime to the ridiculous:

Myth: *"Milk is nature's perfect food. You can be healthy on it alone."*

Fact: Of course not. Persons who believe this might very well develop iron-deficiency anemia, since milk is low in iron. The calcium you would get from living on milk alone would interfere with iron absorption. As we said, milk is a good food, but not the only one you need.

Since we are talking about dairy products, here's a good one about yogurt:

Myth: *"The Hunzas who live to be over 100 eat primarily yogurt and apricots. We will be healthier and live longer if we do the same."*

Fact: A diet that works well for one group of people is not necessarily appropriate for others. You also need to take into account the American "stress factor"—you know, where everyone's running around beating the clock. Other people also exercise more than Americans and generally take better care of their bodies. Once again, the answer lies in nutritional balance and in adjusting diet to meet individual needs.

Myth: *"Vegetarians are better athletes and are healthier than meat eaters."*

Fact: Not so. It is the overall balance of nutrients, rather than their source, that is important. The person who eats meat, fish, and poultry is not less healthy, although we encourage using less of these foods. A vegetarian diet is high in fiber, and unless one eats large amounts of cheese, low in fat.

Myth: *"Herbs are natural and will not cause side effects like prescription medications will. If they don't do what is expected, at least taking them won't do any harm."*

Fact: A physician friend of ours once said, "Poison ivy is natural too, but I wouldn't go rolling around in it!" Many medications in common use originally came from herbs, and using herbs without understanding their medicinal properties can be very harmful. Valarian is a good example. This herb is a sedative and muscle relaxant. Valarian is potentially addicting and not safe for recovering persons.

There are a number of "magic wands" to be broken concerning sugar. Here are three:

Myth: *"Sugar is a white poison that causes many of our major illnesses. Honey, turbinado sugar, and molasses are better."*

Fact: Too much of anything is not good for you, including sugar. It doesn't matter whether it's refined by bees or people. Honey, turbinado or raw sugar, and molasses contain very small amounts of trace minerals but not enough to contribute significant amounts to your diet. Use whatever sweetener you choose in minimal amounts.

Myth: "Candy gives quick energy, so it is the ideal between-meal snack."

Fact: Sure, eating candy will give you a quick energy fix because it raises your blood sugar level quickly, providing you with a sense of well-being. But since you are raising it quickly with sugar, it also drops rapidly, producing a short-lived "high" that requires another candy "fix." You are far better off using fruits, vegetables, whole grains, or yogurt. These are nutrient-dense, low-calorie snacks that make great between-meal snacks.

Myth: "Blackstrap molasses will strengthen the heart because it is high in potassium."

Fact: Blackstrap molasses is a "Catch-22" kind of food. It does contain more minerals because it is what remains after the sugar has been removed and purified. However, blackstrap molasses is a laxative and tends to promote potassium loss rather than absorption. It's quite true that potassium is necessary for a regular heartbeat, but extra potassium does nothing to strengthen it.

Myth: "Brand A vegetable oil is superior to Brand B because it contains no cholesterol."

Fact: No vegetable oil contains cholesterol. Saturated fats such as coconut and palm kernel oil, shortening, and hard margarine encourage the body to make cholesterol. But see how the advertising of brands might lead you to believe that one is better than another because it has "no cholesterol."

Now for all of you who have taken the "grapefruit diet" to heart, this is for you:

Myth: "Grapefruit burns fat and eating it three times a day will ensure weight loss with no effort on your part."

Fact: No food burns fat or increases metabolic rate. Weight loss is brought about by cutting down on the number of calories you consume, exercising regularly, and living a different lifestyle—a lifestyle that doesn't contribute to obesity.

Here are two myths for the "muscle beach" gang:

Myth: *"Muscle cramps during or after exercise are caused by insufficient salt."*

Fact: Muscle cramps result from the loss of large amounts of water through perspiration during strenuous exercise. Want to prevent cramps? Drink water before, during, and after exercise. Salt tablets may make the situation worse.

Myth: *"Protein makes muscles strong. If you are body building or exercising regularly, you'll need to eat large amounts of protein."*

Fact: Once muscles are present, carbohydrates for energy maintain them. You need enough protein to replace lost cells and to maintain your body, but large amounts are not needed. Eating large amounts of protein or purified amino acids hasn't been proven to enhance muscle production. What it does do is build the size of the pockets of the supplement salespeople.

Myth: *"Brewer's yeast in large amounts reverses liver damage."*

Fact: The truth is, nutritional or brewer's yeast is a good source of B-complex vitamins and nothing more. Save your money!

Myth: *"If you use lecithin, you can lower cholesterol by liquefying it."*

Fact: Lecithin is used by commercial food producers to emulsify the fat in salad dressings, ice cream, and candy. But we have no evidence that it will do the same in your bloodstream.

Myth: *"Using medications to remove minerals from the body will slow aging and relieve the symptoms associated with aging."*

Fact: This process is called chelation therapy and is approved for persons who have heavy metal poisoning, but not for other purposes. Unless the person administering this process is very precise, the result is likely to be permanent damage or even death. It sounds like a good idea to remove minerals, especially calcium, from the walls of hardened blood vessels, but the use of this therapy to reverse the process of aging is questionable.

And speaking of aging:

Myth: *"Using nucleic acids will prevent degenerative diseases like cancer and will reverse the aging process."*

Fact: Well we wish it were true, but it isn't. These substances, found in the nucleus of body cells, have not been proven to have any effect on the aging process. You see, nucleic acids are proteins, and as such they are digested and used like any other protein in your body.

Myth: *"If you eat a meal containing different types of foods, it places an extra load on the body. The digestive enzymes of the body are designed to process only certain items. Therefore you should eat foods in a certain order or use only certain combinations of foods."*

Fact: Well, a few people might be helped by eating specific food combinations, but these would be people who have problems digesting food. Nutrients are absorbed better when they are made available slowly, as in the course of a mixed meal. As we mentioned in another chapter, amino acids in purified state overload the system. Since they cannot be absorbed quickly, they are excreted.

After all, eating food is a social, psychological, and emotional experience. If we had to regiment ourselves as the myth suggests, then we would lose much of the pleasure of eating.

Myth: *"Most people have years of accumulated feces in their bodies that need to be removed so that they can properly absorb the nutrients in their food.'*

Fact: For most people a high-fiber diet provides all the intestinal cleansing needed. Besides, most of our food isn't processed in the colon or large intestine. The majority of the processing, and absorption of nutrients, occurs in the small intestine. Now, if someone has had chronic constipation for many years, or perhaps a blocked bowel, then it's possible that medical intervention, including surgery, might be necessary.

And speaking of "cleansing" the body:

Myth: *"Fasting on a regular basis will cleanse the body so that it is prepared to absorb and utilize nutrients more efficiently."*

Fact: Long periods of fasting, especially for recovering persons, are not advisable because of the fluctuation of blood sugar levels. Of course, fasting has long been a part of religious practices. Short fasts might even increase the sense of well-being for some people. In general, however, a healthy body cleanses itself, and fasts or special cleansing programs are not necessary.

Well, there you have it. We have tried to pull some rabbits out of the hat and show you that these myths about food, vitamins, and supplements are just part of a great magic show. Recovering people like to share their experiences of things that "really work" for them. The rest of the population does the same. However, good health, good living, and, above all, solid recovery are based on sticking with the tried and true plans for good eating and good food preparation.

Check facts with a qualified nutritionist and, of course, your physician, before embarking on some new scheme to lose weight or modify your body's chemistry to produce the quick results you saw advertised. If some new idea sounds "too good to be true," the chances are, it *is*. Break the magic wand and get back to hard work in the exercise room and in the kitchen.

PART 2: MAKING THE CHANGES

5
Eating Well Is Part of Loving Yourself

"Are you tired of being a 97-pound weakling?"
"I lost fifteen pounds in just two weeks!"
"You'll never be afraid of looking in the mirror again!"

Wow! Does it bring back memories? Seeing that "puny" little kid who's afraid to go to the beach because he has "no body"? But wait. There's hope! Send away for the "amazing plan" in this offer, and you too can begin to feel better about the way you look.

And off you go on another quick cure to improve the outward appearance that we place such importance upon in our lives. As a recovering person, you'll be particularly sensitive about the excess baggage you acquired while you were drinking.

There is no question that looking good is one of the big payoffs to a life of sobriety. How many times have people said to the person no longer in the battle with alcohol, "Boy, do *you* look great!" It's a super feeling,

60

because you have spent hundreds of hours looking into your bathroom or bedroom mirror on the "morning after" and vowing "never to do it again," only to be lied to again by the image that is reflected back at you. The truth of the matter is, you really *didn't care about yourself.*

What you cared about most was where the next drink was coming from and under what circumstances it was going to be consumed. You know—which particular party, function, or small tête-à-tête would offer the next opportunity for you to get blasted.

When you left for the evening, you thought you looked pretty good—hair in place, makeup on straight, no runs in your stockings, and no stains on the front of your sport coat. That was all you needed: the *outward* appearance that everything was fine with you.

Inside, you were a mess before you even started. By the time another night of drinking was concluded, you had probably vowed to "make a new start" and never do this to yourself again. But you did do it again, until finally you reached whatever crisis led you into treatment and/or the Fellowship of A.A.

Eating well is not only a necessary function in your life, but also a definite stage in the psychological framework of recovery, the stage when you can say, "I'm an OK person, and I'm beginning to like myself!"

What you haven't done up to this point in recovery is to be bold enough to begin loving yourself. But this is an absolutely essential ingredient of recovery. Why? Because if you do not love yourself and the new person that you are trying to become, then it's pretty obvious that you won't be able to offer much love to anyone else.

When you were in the prime of your drinking, eating was probably the last thing on your mind. Oh, you went through the motions alright, but you hardly ever focused your attention on the food that was available. Rather, you were intrigued with the quality and quantity of booze available.

Do you remember all the elaborate dinners that you prepared only to be unable to make it to the table at all or to find yourself just picking at things? Or how about all your good intentions of eating and not drinking as much as usual?

We all know what happened to those great plans, don't we? Essentially, food isn't really a big priority in the active drinker's life. You didn't really care about yourself, much less love yourself. Eating was simply something that you knew had to be done, and in too many cases it was simply an excuse for the drinking that was involved with the eating.

So what we're after here is to get you to understand the link between eating well and loving yourself. In his fine and popular book, *The Road Less Traveled*, Dr. M. Scott Peck says a lot about love and loving yourself. Dr. Peck writes, "When we love ourselves, we attend to our own growth."

The very act of recovery is a message to the world that you love and care about yourself, so much so that you are willing to stop your destructive behavior and get the help necessary to straighten up and fly right.

As you get further into the process of recovery, you begin growth: a personal commitment to make things better for yourself and those who love you. Your drinking was an expression of self-hatred. The same can be said of the junk food that may have become a part of your everyday living. When you aren't paying attention to what you are eating and how you are eating, you are being self-destructive and hateful to yourself, instead of loving.

We are certainly not suggesting that all junk foods are your enemies. The authors (or one of them at least) have certainly been known to consume more than their share of less-than-nutritious food. It's when this kind of food becomes the main course of your daily diet that you are giving a clear message to your body that you don't care a whole lot about it. On the other hand, when you are eating well, you are reinforcing the idea that you are interested in turning your life around and experiencing the joy of being sober.

The truth is that during your active drinking days the whole idea of eating well just didn't have any priority. The compulsion to drink and to continue drinking far outweighed the need to feel good about yourself or to love yourself. Why? Because the alcohol supplied all the love you needed. At least that's the way it seemed. So the idea of really looking good in the clothes you were wearing or of keeping in shape was pushed to the back of your brain, replaced by thoughts of how dynamite you were on the social scene, especially after a "little drink or two."

Let's look at that dynamic for just a moment. When it was necessary for alcohol to play the important role of "breaking the ice" for the usually shy, reserved, quiet man or woman, then alcohol became the dominant factor for continuing to be at ease in social situations that normally caused anxiety and tension.

Go back if you can and look at photographs of yourself taken at a "drinking event," such as a wedding reception or birthday party. Would you really be comfortable looking that way again? Forget the particular hairstyles or skirt lengths of the time, look at *you*. Are you looking out from that photograph like someone who loves himself? Doubtful. Very doubtful!

Instead you are probably seeing someone who was already overweight and wearing a lot of dark clothes to hide the extra pounds. You probably don't have a lot of pictures of yourself in swim wear, since those items of clothing are just too revealing.

Here's another question for you to ponder: how many times did you actually punish yourself by not eating properly? Yes, *punish!* If you had a night of heavy drinking you rarely thought of fighting the resultant hangover by eating three good, well-balanced meals. Rather you would say things like, "God! The *thought* of food makes me sick!" or "If I even *look* at food, I just *know* I'll throw up!"

Of course, what you really knew would fix you up was a "little hair of the dog," namely, a drink or two. This notion comes down to us from the old Latin phrase *Similar similibus curantur*, which tells us that the burnt hair of a dog is the best antidote to its bite.

Well, maybe you thought that a couple of drinks would really help your hangover, but is that a good way of expressing self-love? Today, in recovery, you can and want to be a part of the "wellness scene" because it tells you and those around you that you have begun to care about yourself again. The destructive forces that were at work with alcohol abuse have been replaced, we hope, by a program of recovery in which you may be engaging in regular exercise (see Chapter 12), counting your calories and watching your cholesterol intake, and generally rediscovering what good, nutritious eating is all about.

When this wonderful feeling begins to take hold of you, then you are beginning the very important process of transferring your old love of alcohol to the love of yourself as a new, whole, and giving person. It's exciting and you deserve it! Why? Because this feeling is one of the payoffs to sobriety.

We all need some payoff or reward for our efforts. The mere act of drinking alcohol was in itself a payoff, one that was instantly available. When you felt bad, you took a little drink and started to "feel good." This behavior was reinforced over and over.

Now that sobriety is your priority, where's the payoff? Well, there are many, but one of them certainly is your newfound enjoyment of the food you eat, how it's prepared and served. An added payoff is the way in which you can now sit down to enjoy a meal in casual, unhurried mouthfuls.

When you drink, the food you consume doesn't really have a lot of taste in spite of the number of times you may have sworn that beer and pizza go together or that red wine and spaghetti are inseparable.

But now food has the flavor and the aroma that were all but masked by the taste and the smell of the alcohol you were consuming. It's a real pleasure to be able to sit down to a well-prepared meal and to be able to enjoy it. Eating responsibly and appreciatively is its own reward, part of loving yourself.

So we can look at ourselves, even critically, and realize that there are some changes we would like to make, once we have alcohol out of our lives. The fact that we want to make those changes is healthy, and the act of doing something about how we eat, what we eat, and how much we eat is all part of loving the new self that comes from living life without alcohol.

We'll be talking about how and what to eat throughout this book. Find out how good you can feel and look. Your self-esteem and your eating habits have a lot to do with each other. Bon appétit!

6
Make the Changes!
Take the Heat!

When you begin to make changes, you're going to take some heat from your family. No doubt about it. We're talking about the heat that you take from family and friends when you decide to make changes anywhere in your lifestyle, but mostly when food is involved. We are such creatures of habit (when it comes to food, anyway) that when you try and depart from the way things "are supposed to be," you can really get into trouble.

Well, recovery means making changes of all kinds, and since this is a book about how eating habits affect your life, in this chapter we're going to help you make some real changes that will—well, yes—be good for you.

Even if you live alone, changing your food choices and eating habits affects the way you interact with others. Others may feel threatened when you try to kick the junk-food habit, for example.

Your refusal of rich desserts means you are taking care of yourself, but frequently family, friends, and

significant others react with guilt. They express this
guilt by attacking you for being on some "crazy diet" or
for "trying to be better than we are!"

Some of the people you thought were your friends
may suddenly not want to associate with you, the new
you who likes taking care of yourself. When you were
actively drinking, you were living on the brink of
mental and physical disaster. You totally disregarded
the health risks associated with the typical American
diet, in addition to filling your body with booze on a
regular basis. Not good at all!

So now, part of your recovery plan definitely involves
making some unpopular changes in your eating habits.
Oh, there will be pressure to revert to the old ways.
Whether you share a restaurant meal or accept an
invitation to someone's home for a meal, you're going to
be subjected to a lot of pressure to return to the old,
unhealthy way of doing things.

But making changes is such an important part of
recovery that you need to have the courage to just go
ahead and turn a deaf ear to the criticism. Do what
you've got to do. No one else is going to get hurt. Your
example may even inspire a friend or two, but take care
of yourself first and let the others tag along if they
choose.

Some facts about the role of food in our lives, other
than as a source of nutrition, might help you over a few
of the rougher spots ahead. One of our first experiences
after birth is being fed. When a baby is being fed, a lot
of information about food and the attitudes toward it is
being transmitted, communicated through the senses
from mother (or other caretaker) to child.

The way an infant is held, talked to, looked at,
"cooed" over, etc., help communicate whether or not
the caretaker loves, cares for, enjoys, and wants the
baby. It also communicates the caretaker's enjoyment
of food. Well, all of that helps us as babies to relate
emotionally, not just intellectually, to food and the

eating experience. Changing lifelong, ingrained habits is difficult, to say the least. It certainly is as difficult as changing individual foods themselves, but change you must!

We are certainly not suggesting that you can recover from the disease of alcoholism by changing how and what you eat. Food is one part of the total effort a person makes on the path to recovery. As we have said and will continue to say throughout this book, you do not pay a great deal of attention to anything in your life (including food and eating habits) while you are in the active drinking stage. Now, it's time to start some radical thinking for the new you.

Some people are changing their diets as an essential part of recovery and/or improvement of physical health. These people are so highly motivated that they have very little or no problem in making a total change seemingly overnight. Other people believe that changing their diet is disruptive and even life-threatening. Their attitude says, "I've survived on this diet, and changing it is going to kill me!"

Some other people consider these changes to be mere stepping-stones toward a greater goal and therefore see them as temporary. For this group of people, the changes in diet will remain in effect until they have achieved the desired weight loss or until their cholesterol level or sugar levels drop. Then they go back to their old ways. This keeps them on a merry-go-round of on-again, off-again dieting. Nuts to that!

Unfortunately, most of us experience some or all of these feelings and tend to resist change, even denying the need to make changes. Then a strange thing happens. We start to accept the need to change and then get angry about it. We feel deprived. We may even start to bargain with ourselves, telling ourselves that we will keep to this diet only until we "get better," and then we can return to our old ways. This makes as much sense as believing that alcoholics can return to some magical kind of "controlled" drinking. Not so.

Fortunately, most recovering alcoholics learn to accept that their bodies have certain nutritional needs that differ from those of the average person. In addition, these same people become aware that dietary changes are not temporary, but essential aspects of the total recovery process. Recovery is a lot more than just quitting drinking. Recovery means being as healthy as possible in all aspects of your life.

Now let's dispel one myth right here. Eating well does not mean that you have to turn into some kind of "health-food nut." Foods that are high in nutritional value can be purchased right in your friendly neighborhood supermarket or in your favorite restaurants. They don't require special preparation techniques, unusual equipment, or even extra preparation time, once their use is understood.

What you might end up doing is spending some extra time at the beginning reading labels and studying the various ingredients. We'll urge you to cook with less salt, sugar, and fat and avoid foods that are high in these ingredients. Well, this obviously means that a lot of convenience foods are going to be off limits to you.

Because we will be asking you to eliminate some sauces and gourmet-type dishes, you may feel your new diet will be boring. But don't give up! Different doesn't necessarily mean bad. You will be disappointed, however, if you look for substitutes for your old favorites.

Different foods with new flavors and textures add interest and variety. They will increase your enjoyment, rather than limit it. This is going to be a gradual process, just like the rest of your recovery. Making sudden changes isn't recommended. For goodness' sake, don't be like the person we know who attended a nutritional seminar, then went home and stripped the kitchen of all foods that weren't "healthy."

You know what happened then, don't you? The teenagers in the household were summoned and told that from now on they would all be eating a macrobiotic vegetarian diet. Well, the battle started right with that announcement. The kids refused to eat anything until their hot dogs and potato chips were restored.

Those teenagers aren't alone, of course. Very few of us like to have our routines disrupted, especially when it comes to food habits. Even when we are convinced that the change might be in our best interest many of us will feel deprived and cheated if we cannot have our favorite candy, ice cream, or cookies. When we have these feelings, we may find ourselves sneaking around for those special foods or, worse yet, gorging on them and then feeling guilty because we didn't eat right.

Part of your decision will be based on your ability to organize your priorities. Choose one thing and then implement it slowly. Let's take the simple example of, say, brown rice. You can start mixing in a little brown rice with your usual white rice. Don't suddenly switch over to brown rice only. Give yourself and everyone else a chance to become familiar with and appreciate the chewy texture of brown rice.

How about this one? Add a small amount of leaf lettuce to your usual head lettuce. This will permit you to adapt gradually to the difference in texture and flavor. Family members who may not be undergoing the process of recovery may need a little longer to make these changes; their motivation probably isn't as strong as yours. But stick with it!

Kids, as everyone knows, are particularly resistant to change after the age of 18 months. They have their own ideas about what does and does not constitute good food. Young children can get pretty vocal about their food and raise a ruckus when asked to try new things. Others have more adventurous natures and take to new things readily.

Involve your children in the food selection and preparation to help them accept change more easily.

A SMOOTH TRANSITION

So, let's look at some eating habits that often need

changing and suggest ways to implement these changes on a gradual basis. We'll return to our old standbys, the basic food groups, and leave any decision as to their importance in your diet up to you. That is, you decide what will have the greatest impact on your well-being, and then make the changes one at a time. Now here's the hooker in the plan. Once you and your family have become accustomed to the change, go on to another one. A journey of a thousand miles, remember, is made one step at a time. So, here we go!

Fruits and Vegetables

This is the most frequently neglected group of foods. The simplest and most basic change that could be made is to just include more of them in your diet. You might consider some of these suggestions:

- Serve carrot and celery sticks and cherry tomatoes with a dip made of blended yogurt, cottage cheese, and herbs before dinner as an appetizer.
- Mix vegetables into familiar casseroles that are already well liked.
- Add small amounts of an unfamiliar vegetable to a familiar dish.
- In addition to the regular iceberg lettuce in a salad, start using a wide variety of raw vegetables. These will add color to the salad, and you can use your creative talents to make attractive combinations.
- Make fruit salad with fresh, canned, or frozen fruits for dessert. You can top fruit salad with small amounts of coconut or chopped nuts to make it more special.
- Blend fruit and vanilla yogurt to make a quick fruit pudding.
- Start making a fresh fruit bowl instead of the usual cookies and candies that are now being used for snacks.
- Drink fruit juice instead of soda. If you want

carbonation, mix the juice with seltzer or sparkling water.

Cereals and Grains

Here your goal should be to eat more whole grains and fewer refined grains. Try these changes (one at a time, remember!):

- Substitute cracked-wheat bread for white. As family members become accustomed to it, gradually increase the percentage used. Once everyone is happy with cracked-wheat bread, start using 100 percent whole-wheat bread occasionally. Gradually increase the amount used. Sometimes this can take a long time to accomplish, sometimes you can make the switch overnight.
- Substitute whole-wheat flour for part of the flour in a recipe. This will help everyone to learn to like the different texture and flavor of the whole wheat. It's a little drier than white, so you'll need a little more liquid when you use it.
- Mix a little brown rice into the white rice you prepare and gradually increase the proportion added.
- Mix a small amount of a hot whole-wheat cereal with farina.
- Use long-cooking oats instead of the quick oats. You're only adding 2 minutes of cooking time, anyhow.

Dairy Products

As you know, these foods contain saturated fat and should not be consumed in large quantities if cholesterol levels are high. In addition, fat is the most concentrated source of calories; reducing your intake of dairy products helps keep calories down. Here are some ideas for those who don't include enough dairy foods in their diets.

- Try using 2 percent milk instead of whole milk, which contains 3½ to 4 percent fat. Once this has been accepted, switch to 1 percent or skim milk.
- Substitute low-fat cheese for regular. Mozzarella is a skim-milk cheese (check the label to make sure). Cheese that is labeled "partially skim-milk cheese" is made with a mixture of skim milk and cream and thus has the same fat content as full-fat cheese. It is another good transition food on the way to skim milk or low-fat cheese.
- Extra powdered milk can be added to muffins, biscuits, and those Sunday-morning pancakes.
- Low-fat plain yogurt can be used in recipes calling for sour cream. The flavor is similar, but the calories are reduced by about two-thirds. Yogurt makes a great topping for baked potatoes when chives and garlic powder are added. Substitute it for mayonnaise in salad dressings. Add a few drops of vanilla and frozen concentrated fruit juice and you have a great dessert topping.

Meat, Fish, Poultry, and Eggs

Most people eat far more from this group than they should. These foods are, as discussed earlier, the primary sources of protein, and they're also high in fat. So one suggestion for a change in diet is to reduce the amount you eat from this group. Other suggestions:

- Trim all visible fat before cooking.
- Bake, broil, or stew meat and poultry. Bake, steam, and poach fish.
- Use tomato sauce, yogurt, and/or herbs and spices for seasoning instead of breading, frying, and cooking in sauces high in fat.

- Reduce serving sizes to 2-to-3-ounce portions twice a day, and get your other calories from grains, bread, potatoes, and other starchy vegetables.
- Emphasize poultry and fish. This reduces the intake of saturated fats.
- Include salmon, mackerel, cod, red snapper, and tuna once or twice a week to supply fatty acids that help reduce cholesterol.

Seasonings

These items are all overused. So our concern is to help you reduce the amounts of sugar, salt, fats, and oils that you consume. Here are some ideas.

- Decrease the amount of sugar and salt in a recipe by one-fourth. When the flavor of the food seems acceptable, reduce it by another fourth. Most of us can learn to really like food with half the amount of sugar and salt called for in the recipe.
- Purchase canned fruit packed in juice rather than syrup, or get dry-pack frozen fruit. You might need to start by using fruit in a light syrup and gradually work your way into the juice-packed fruits.
- Look for frozen or canned vegetables with less salt and no sugar. Avoid frozen vegetables with sauces.
- Keep eating foods without using sugar or salt. Get to know and like the natural flavor of foods.
- Experiment with herbs and spices that enhance the natural flavor of foods.
- Have fresh fruit for dessert instead of sugary baked desserts.
- Mix butter and oil together (1 stick of butter and ½ cup oil) to make a soft spread that can be used in smaller amounts and then refrigerated.
- Serve cooked vegetables with little or no butter or oil added for seasoning.

- Add extra vinegar or lemon juice to salad dressings to dilute the oil, or use no-oil salad dressings.

In addition to being aware of how food affects your interactions with family and friends, you need to recognize that when you change your eating habits, you may experience some emotional ups and downs.

These feelings might be the result of changes in your biochemistry accompanying your change in diet. You might experience a feeling of deprivation. In this case, you are probably making too many changes too fast. These changes may make you feel that another of life's pleasures (drinking was one, too) is being denied to you.

Setting your own personal goals and making your dietary changes gradually will pay off for you as you take the time to love yourself by eating well. Food functions as a sort of "ice breaker" or a "social lubricant" in our society. It is more than a source of vitamins, minerals, and calories; eating is also a social experience. When you eat frequently in the company of others, you might have to look at the changes you are trying to make and come up with food goals that don't offend people. In other words, you will have to learn to be comfortable turning down a rich dessert or sticking to your guns when your friend says, "You can go off your diet just this once!"

The siren songs of "I made it especially for you" and "I'll be so hurt if you don't eat this" need to be tactfully ignored and answered with songs of your own that tell you to be strong and stick to your dietary changes.

You are going to take some heat. But this business of recovery requires that you place a great deal of trust in the process. These changes in eating habits may not win you any popularity contests at the outset. But hang in there. You (and your family or other loved ones) will be the eventual winners.

7
Diets Don't Work

"No, thanks! I'm on a diet."
"See that size 8? That's what I'm shooting for!"
"Pie? Not a chance! Wanna wreck my diet?"

Oh, boy! We Americans are a vain bunch, aren't we? When you have to let your belt out another notch, or the scales start singing to you in the "upper notes," wham! you go on a diet. You need to take the weight off yesterday. Fast-weight-loss diets abound, and the chances are you've given most of them a shot. Last year's or last month's didn't work as well as you thought, though. There wasn't enough instant gratification, so you abandoned it and are moving on to the next.

Since this new diet worked so well for your friend, you think you'll probably give it a try, too. Being thin is in. So what'll it be this time? High protein, low carbohydrate? How about just dieting all week and then eating anything and everything on the weekends? You can hit the fiber trail so you always feel full. How about "weight-loss tea" from Japan? After all, except for a few Sumo wrestlers, have you seen a lot of fat Japanese? It must work.

Herbs are good for you, so why not try the herbal diet your neighbor is selling? Of course you don't have time for exercise, so you need something that doesn't involve aerobics, swimming, jogging, or bike riding. Maybe you could just get a pill that would curb your appetite so that you would stop eating when you should and you wouldn't have to bother looking for special foods. So you're stuck with the old bottom line, if you'll excuse the pun. If you want to drop 25 pounds, you begin searching for something that will make the least demand on your time and energy.

You probably give little or no thought to how this diet food or drink will taste, how much it costs, or how it might affect your health. Now 'fess up! Didn't your last diet start on a Monday, so that you could spend the weekend loading up on desserts, fried foods, sauces, breads, and potatoes with gravy? Sure you did! We call this a "diet mentality" and it's the common denominator in what has been called "America's favorite indoor sport"—dieting!

If you have chosen one of the popular quick-weight-loss diets that guarantees you'll take off 29 pounds the first month (or double your money back), the food formula you are eating is not the regular food to which you are accustomed. You assume that once you reach your weight goal, you can return to your old eating habits and still maintain your new svelte look. But oh, the pain!

After a day or two, maybe a week, you start feeling deprived, so you decide one little treat won't hurt. Then the dynamics of "one little taste won't hurt" or "I made this specially for you!" go to work, and woosh! the plan ends up in the wastebasket after two to three weeks at the most.

You can't ignore social pressure around foods. Eating

is a social experience, and through the food choices we make, we communicate who we are and what we think of ourselves. Food is often used to manipulate. If you turn down food that has been offered as a means of, say, establishing intimacy, then you are not just rejecting the food, but rejecting the giver as well. No wonder folks act as if their own little world had collapsed if you have the courage to say no and really stick to it. You have flat outright said no to them! Let's not even talk about those hurt feelings.

So what does happen when you diet? That is, what are the physical and psychological changes that occur? The first thing you lose is water—3 to 10 pounds of it the first week. Then your metabolism changes, that is, the rate at which calories are used. The metabolic rate drops, and every calorie is used as efficiently as possible. After a while, your body gets so good at adapting that it can gain or at least maintain weight on 800 calories a day. Your body doesn't differentiate between actual starvation and drastic dieting to look fashionably beautiful.

Your brain gets into the act really quickly as it begins to convert protein into the vital glucose that it needs. Converting protein into glucose is easier than converting fat. Since you have cut down on carbohydrates, your body goes to work on the available protein. The result? You begin to lose muscle. If you go to extremes, you will lose organ tissue. Now here's the real killer! If weight loss from muscle and organ tissue really continued at the rate promised in those diet ads, you wouldn't be around for more than three weeks.

Fortunately, our bodies are very adaptable and don't give up that easily. Body fat reserves are converted into usable energy, but not in the usual way. You see, fat cannot be easily used for energy unless some carbohydrate is available. The fat partially breaks down into its component parts, stopping at a substance we have talked about before, ketones. Half your brain cells can adapt to using ketones for energy, even though it's a substitute "fuel." Ketones suppress appetite and for a while you feel good, even "high." Remember when we were talking about ketones and running? Same thing.

Then comes the revolution. About three to seven days into the dieting process, the body begins to scream at you. Thought processes may slow down, mood swings become more extreme, and you may fly off the handle when you least expect it.

Ketones disrupt the balance of specialized minerals, minerals that regulate heartbeat and are also responsible for transmitting messages. When this disruption occurs, you may suffer irregular heartbeat and/or muscle spasms. When this reaction to the ketones occurs, we say a person is in a state of ketosis. A lot of people have told us they find it more dangerous to ride in a car with someone in a state of ketosis than with someone who has had too much to drink. Another sure sign of ketosis is bad breath. Quick-weight-loss "experts" will stress the importance of getting "into ketosis," so that you can tell that body fat is being lost. They will take urine samples to check for ketones. Very few of these people will talk about the inherent dangers of ketosis.

As we said earlier, your body doesn't recognize the difference between being starved for the sake of beauty and being starved to death. Your body just starts doing whatever it takes to survive.

The plan your body puts into action calls for lowering the metabolic rate and then making the best possible use of every calorie available. It's like an NFL coach looking to his full squad, including those on "injured reserve," to get the game won.

If this is your first go-around with a quick-weight-loss diet, then your body doesn't catch on as quickly to what's happening, and the chances are good that you'll lose the weight, just like the book or plan promised. But look out if this is the tenth time you've tried this kind of diet.

Your body will adapt in a matter of days, and the promised weight loss won't happen. So you counter-react and try to reduce your calories some more. Again you body adapts, keeping one or two steps ahead of you. Now your frustration really increases. No matter how little you eat, you don't "budge from your bulge." You just maintain your present weight. When your frustration reaches its peak, you decide you might as well eat because "this diet is no good anyway."

Your metabolic rate is still low at this point, and calories are being used very efficiently. End result? You gain back all the weight you lost, plus 5 to 10 pounds more. This "yo-yo" effect of "putting it on" and "taking it off" makes you mad, and being mad doesn't help you recognize that what took years to put on will take time to get off. The pattern will continue until you under-stand the process.

Just like your sobriety, losing weight and keeping it off requires time, commitment, energy, and a change in lifestyle. You have already learned that you can live your life quite successfully without alcohol and drugs, but you cannot survive long without food.

The appeal of these fad diets is that the change they require of you is temporary. After the diet, you think you can return to your old habits. Well, if that worked, it would be ideal, but the fact is that a temporary change of diet is just like temporary sobriety or offer-ing an alcoholic a "controlled drinking" situation. It doesn't work.

Your eating patterns were established before you learned to talk, and so you relate to food emotionally rather than intellectually. You might know on an intel-lectual level what needs to be changed, but internaliz-ing the change, making it a part of your life, is a highly charged, emotional experience. It takes roughly twice as long to establish and maintain new dietary habits. If the consequence of breaking the diet is physical pain, occurring within 24 hours, then the change will be made more easily. But when you're dealing with losing weight and all the social complications involved, change is harder.

If you can stay with a dietary change for a period of six months, then it is pretty well established. You have to be careful, though. Breaking the diet for just one sliver of pie might be OK, but if you then add just one sliver of cake, a candy bar, and an ice cream cone, then you're in for a relapse. You'll be off and running again on a rich, high-calorie diet, and you'll be eating this way regularly and compulsively. If you're really interested in a healthy diet that is low in calories, coupled with a change in lifestyle, then plan on spending at least one year to establish your new habits to the point that you feel comfortable with them.

Now let's look at a few points that will help you achieve and maintain your desired weight. Call them guidelines for a new dietary lifestyle.

- *Put weight in its proper perspective.* If your parents are of stocky build, the chances of your getting to be slim and willowy aren't very good. So instead of trying to look like the model on the cover of *Vogue*, assess your attributes and then decide on a realistic weight goal based on your height and body build. What you're trying to avoid is raising your stress level. A weight you can reach but not maintain without constantly keeping your guard up is just going to take the fun out of living.
- *Don't lose for special occasions* or for someone else. Don't try and take off weight for the holidays or that "dream vacation." This just increases your stress load and sets you up for failure.

- *Put food in its proper perspective* as a source of essential nutrients and as an enjoyable social experience. Eat for your well-being, not because:
  1. It's a reward.
  2. People are starving in the world.
  3. Your friends insist you eat.
  4. It's time to eat.
  5. You're a member of the "clean plate" club.
  6. There might not be any food later.
  7. You're bored, mad, sad, angry, or scared.
  8. You might not be in Hawaii, Dallas, New York, etc., again.
  9. You are procrastinating.
  10. Someone else paid for it.
- *Examine why* it might be comfortable for you to stay at your present weight. You might not want to lose weight because it would bring you emotionally and physically closer to people. It might make people relate to you on the basis of looks rather than because they like you.
- *Keep a chart of what you eat*—when, where, and why—for one week. Most people have eating habits that follow specific patterns. Binges and periods of high-calorie-food consumption are likely to occur at regular intervals in the day, week, or month. Be honest.
- *Be aware of your body's hunger signals* and eat only when you are truly hungry. Most overweight persons don't know what hunger feels like; some will have to go without food for a long time before feeling hunger.
- *Consume 1,200 calories a day,* or at least make that your goal. If you're under a physician's care for weight loss, or you're under 5 feet tall, you can get by on less. The idea here is to supply less than your body needs to maintain weight, but enough to provide essential nutrients and to prevent starvation from setting in.

Each pound of body fat stores 3,500 calories. In

theory then, a pound a week can be lost by reducing your calorie intake by 500 calories per day. However we know this does not work for everyone. We do know that rapid weight loss is usually due to loss of water and some lean muscle.

In order to lose body fat and maintain muscle, weight loss must be restricted to one to two pounds a week on the average. Warning: if you find yourself obsessed with food, your calorie intake is too low. Remember, too, that weight loss occurs in a "stair-step" fashion. That is, you'll lose a few pounds and then plateau for a while. This is your body's way of adjusting to change. If you stay on a plateau for more than two weeks, then adjustments need to be made.

- *Stay off the scale,* or at least don't weigh yourself every day. Your weight may vary by 2 to 3 pounds in a 24-hour period. Climbing on the scales every morning is going to affect your mood for the whole day. Weigh yourself once a week and you'll get a better sense of how you're doing.
- *Exercise regularly* to raise your metabolic rate and maintain or increase muscle mass. We recommend aerobic exercise for 20 to 30 minutes a day. Overexercising can do more harm than good by causing muscle loss. Also, if you exercise infrequently or only every other day, you won't increase your metabolic rate as easily as if you were exercising on a daily basis. Your goal is to lose fat, not muscle.
- *Eat only when you are hungry,* but don't go for excessively long periods of time without eating. Skipping meals sets up the body's starvation reactions again. It needs to get the message that food will be supplied on a regular basis. Your primary sources of calories should be fruits, vegetables, and whole grains, all high in carbohydrates. Protein foods such as meat, fish, and poultry contain hidden fat and add unwanted calories.
- *Develop an awareness* of what your body feels like

when you've had enough to eat. Your goal should be to never feel stuffed or completely satisfied. Once you've been able to identify your body's signal and are aware of it after most meals, you can use it as your guide. The lucky folks who maintain their weight without special diets are the people who know this signal well. When they want to lose weight, they just stop eating before the signal is given, or when about four more bites would taste good.

- *Match your eating habits* to your body's needs. If you're a morning person, then breakfast is a very important meal. If you're on the midnight shift, then a heavy meal at night might be in order. Try to maintain regular hours and be consistent. If you work a rotating shift, you may find it difficult to lose weight. Why? Because your body is constantly readjusting to your changing food and exercise patterns.

If you are going out for a special meal that might involve eating more than is on your diet, then eat less before and after the special meal. When you buy snacks and treats for others, get things that you don't like, so you won't be tempted. Saying grace at your table can do more for you than just expressing gratitude for the food you are about to eat. It's a time to focus attention on the way you eat and your attitude toward your food.

Slow down, eat consciously. Don't eat while watching TV, reading, or working. If you can, take your shoes off if you have to eat at your desk. That way your mind won't be wandering on to the next task but will be focused on eating a good meal.

If you're eating in your car, try and pull into a park or rest area where you can eat consciously rather than gobbling a few bites at each traffic light.

- *Don't become a human garbage can*, devouring leftovers, particularly if you can't resist temptation.

Leftovers are just what their name says, something to be used later in a soup or stew if there's more than a tablespoon of it. Otherwise, out in the garbage it goes. Not in *you!*

It may be difficult, but don't socialize in the kitchen. Serve plates in the kitchen and avoid going back for seconds. If you get hungry between meals, drink water. If you are still hungry in half an hour, you can eat a small snack or meal if it's the right time of day. Even the strongest of you may give in to a binge and go off your diet. But don't go on an all-out binge. Get right back on your diet the next meal.

- *Get the "doggie" bag or box first* in a restaurant. Put half your meal in the box before taking the first bite. You can have what's in the box for your next meal. If you try to just eat half, you'll cheat. Or you'll lose track. As we've said before, control your portions of dressings and butter by having them served on the side. Don't order sour cream or gravy, and don't have dessert unless it's fresh fruit.
- *Get involved at parties and social gatherings.* Concentrate on the people and not the food. If necessary, eat a light snack before going to the party and then snack on fresh fruit and vegetables rather than chips and dips. If it's a sit-down function, take small portions. If you are worried about taking too much, eat a small amount before going out so you won't be starved.

  Eat at regular times, and don't skip meals or go too long without eating, because when you're hungry you tend to inhale the food rather than eat it.
- *Don't shop when you're hungry* because those forbidden foods look extra tempting when you've not eaten for a while. By the way, we suggest you avoid diet foods. They usually don't taste as good as regular foods and they encourage the diet mentality that says, "I'm deprived because I must eat in a

special way; therefore I'll binge."

- *Cut down on coffee* and other caffeine products. Caffeine stimulates the appetite and can stimulate the craving for sweets and snacks.

- *Try a hot soup and/or salad* before your entree, particularly if you are dining out. This will help you eat more slowly. You'll eat less of the entree because you'll feel full. Be sure the soup is not a creamed variety, however.

- *Let folks get their own snacks,* and don't you try to supply them! Know why? Sure you do. If they're around, you'll eat them, too. Other family members can prepare their own snacks and you won't be so inclined to sample them or "have just one."

Finally, it's important that you enjoy life and the food that you consume. You can contribute to the good life by making mealtimes enjoyable. Set an attractive table, and allow a few minutes before eating for creating a calm atmosphere. Limit the places you eat in your home to one or two, and establish some new ways of preparing and eating food. Try new recipes (like the ones we've included in the last chapter. Food is important in your life, but it shouldn't be the main focus, so keep it in perspective.

When you plan a weight-loss program, make it *your* responsibility and not that of your spouse, your children, roommate, or friends. When you place *them* in charge of your food habits, you are heading for mutual resentment, surreptitious behavior, and a failed diet.

Just like your sobriety, the commitment to achieving and maintaining your desired weight is a full-time, permanent lifestyle change. The success of any program will depend on your willingness to supply the necessary time, effort, courage, good sense, and attention to the essentials of nutrition that we have introduced to you, perhaps for the first time, in the pages of this book.

8
From One Addiction to Another

*"Good Lord, Brad! That's not just a dish of ice
    cream; that's a barrelfull!"*
*"Charlene, isn't that a lot of coffee for you to be
    drinking?"*
*"I can't keep enough candy in the candy dish.
    He's constantly nibbling at it!"*

Alcoholics have a very neat system that allows them
to trade their addiction to alcohol for another addiction.
And they do a bang-up job of it, too. It's understandable,
isn't it? Once an addictive lifestyle is in place, changing
to another way of thinking and behaving is extremely
difficult.

When the alcohol is out of your system, the patterns
of behavior that made your addiction to it possible
continue to function in your life. So it's easy to replace
the alcohol with candy, cigarettes, coffee, or what have
you.

THE FOOD ADDICTION

It stands to reason that the behavior pattern most

likely to become addictive when you give up alcohol is eating. Why? They both offer immediate gratification. When food is involved, you get a reward (usually a sugary one) by overindulging, so naturally you begin to eat the way you were drinking—to excess and with little or no regard for the consequences.

First of all, there is a "Catch-22" involved here. The people around you are so delighted with your having given up alcohol that they generally ignore the fact that you have traded one addiction for another. We are guilty of encouraging the overeating, particularly in the early stages of treatment and recovery. We have worked at hospital facilities where the refrigerator in the patients' "community room" is jammed with ice cream bars for a while. Soon after treatment is underway and the refrigerator can't be kept full enough anymore, the ice cream begins to be replaced with fruit, carrot sticks, celery, and other vegetables for snacking.

Almost any food can become addictive, particularly, it seems, among recovering persons. A person who feels he or she must have a certain type of food daily and who experiences withdrawal symptoms when it is not available, has a food addiction. For some, this is a psychological reaction to a food that gives comfort in a time of stress.

Physical addiction to a food or to a food group may also be an indicator of an allergy or a food sensitivity. Persons who have this type of reaction exhibit the same behavior patterns as when they were drinking. For example, if you are one of these people, you might feel better and more comfortable when you are eating the particular food. You might experience a real withdrawal when the food is unavailable. You might actually crave the food and feel you cannot go for any length of time without it. Sound familiar? You bet!

You might actually find yourself needing a "fix" of the food just as you did with the booze. Without it you don't feel normal and you develop a drinking behavior, making real efforts to get to the "food of your choice."

Some persons with food sensitivities will crave sugar or carbohydrates. The explanation for this craving seems to relate to hypoglycemia (low blood sugar). These people will be tested and found not to have hypoglycemia at all, but their reactions to the particular food mimic hypoglycemia. These people feel as if their blood sugar level has dropped and so they crave sugar. These symptoms can be relieved by eating a number of small meals and/or consuming high-carbohydrate foods.

To our knowledge, at least, no statistics on the relationship between alcoholism and food sensitivity or chemical sensitivity have been kept, but our own work with recovering patients suggests that between 10 and 20 percent of recovering persons develop food sensitivities or allergies due to alcoholism.

Some allergy specialists believe that somewhere in the family tree of every highly allergic person is at least one alcoholic. Other allergists feel that the presence of alcoholism is coincidental to the allergies. It stands to reason that some recovering persons had allergies before beginning to drink heavily and find that they are worse after sobriety has been achieved. Other people will find that allergies or food sensitivities seem to appear during the recovery process.

Some of the reactions seen are hives, difficult breathing, or headaches. A person may find he is having trouble processing information. Obviously, eliminating the foods that cause problems, or at least using less of them in your daily diet, might relieve these symptoms.

If you are sensitive to certain foods and continue to have problems, it is in your best interest to consult an allergist, a specialist who can help you plan a special diet or perhaps give you allergy shot therapy.

Since being fit and trim is the fashion of the day, the emphasis everywhere is on how we look. This poses a problem for the recovering person who has begun to eat in the same addictive fashion that he or she was drinking. The dilemma: "How to eat all I want and still be thin and in style?" or "Who cares about health or what might happen tomorrow, as long as I can indulge myself today?" So, being typically alcoholic in behavior, you begin to use alcoholic thinking that tells you, "as long as no one sees you gobbling up the candy, cakes, and cookies, it can't possibly be hurting you!"

Now that sounds familiar, doesn't it? And sure enough, off you go to the store to shop for dinner. But in the store, those bags of cookies and those ice cream bars just happen to get broken into, and you begin some addictive eating, namely, you start gorging.

This kind of thinking becomes especially dangerous when it comes to ways of purging ourselves of those unwanted calories that are bound to pile up with this excessive eating.

There are several methods to "purge" extra calories, the most common of which are self-induced vomiting and the use of laxatives, or combinations of the two. The idea is that you can go ahead and indulge yourself, whether in the grocery store, the car, or at a party, and not even think about what is happening to your hips and waistline. You don't have to think about it because you can throw up later, thus regaining control of the situation. Or so you think.

Compulsive eaters tend to be perfectionists, demanding far more of themselves than is humanly possible. Since this is a fact of their addictive behavior, they need a break from this perfectionism. They get that break by eating compulsively—gorging—and losing control.

As in alcoholic drinking, compulsive eaters can experience "blackouts," losing their sense of time and surroundings while gorging. When they realize that they have lost control, panic sets in and they want desperately to be back in control of themselves. So they take laxatives or induce vomiting to get rid of the binge-calories. You can readily see the connection. The substance we are talking about now is food, but the behavior it is provoking is strikingly similar to that of alcohol abuse.

As we've suggested earlier, the foods usually chosen for this type of eating are the "forbidden fruits" of the dieter; all the sweet, greasy treats full of instant gratification are in this category.

Ice cream is also a favorite because the compulsive eater can relieve him or herself by self-induced vomiting. It comes back up as easily as it goes down. Obviously the foods chosen for this type of eating can't take up a lot of time being chewed; that would only delay the gratification. Milk shakes, cream soups, etc., which can be inhaled, are preferred by compulsive eaters.

Consuming food quickly and furtively is part of the addictive pattern. Believe it or not, the idea of possibly getting caught is exciting and enticing to the addictive eater. Sneaking food is the big game.

The ways in which food-sneaking can be done are beyond your wildest imagination. When the urge to gorge comes upon the recovering person, the urge to bypass anything helpful (like talking about your feelings) is overwhelming. Instead you go directly to the food.

Life for the recovering person in the early stages is not as rosy as one would hope for. If it's not easy, the little kid within you may be wanting to act out his frustration by giving himself a treat. Alcohol is out, binge-eating is in, and the addictive behavior goes right on.

Because you may be feeding this "kid" within you, the favorite foods of your childhood tend to be your favorites now. Cookies, candy, and cake, in addition to ice cream, are the obvious choices, with chocolate in almost any form being the all-time favorite "forbidden fruit." There are some chocolate desserts, for example, which almost any compulsive eater will describe as "sensuous." Many of the patients we see will use this term to describe chocolate mousse.

Binge-eating has its own set of strange rules. Foods consumed while driving home from the store, watching TV, reading a favorite book, or studying "don't count" in the calorie department. Another rule tells that "little kid" within you that when the urge to binge starts, it needs to be taken care of right away. Food becomes the "drug of choice," and nothing had better get in your way or slow you down.

"Don't tell me to take care of that kid within me by reading a book," one of our patients loudly stated, "or go for a walk, either! That takes time, and I can stuff cookies in my face for 5 minutes and satisfy myself!"

But once the binge is completed, the need to regain control becomes paramount and thus the induced vomiting or the use of laxatives. Most compulsive eaters are not aware of the fact that even these methods don't get rid of all the calories, only about a third, and that there is a real and present danger in induced vomiting.

The damage caused by vomiting is similar to the damage caused by alcohol. The esophagus was not designed to handle acid and becomes very irritated when it comes in contact with stomach acid. The pressure from vomiting can also cause the rupture of blood vessels in the esophagus, and the stomach acid mentioned earlier has a tendency to etch the enamel on teeth, causing rapid decay and bad breath. Vomiting puts pressure on the glands in your throat, causing bulging, breaking blood vessels in your face, and perhaps causes bags to form under your eyes.

The person practicing self-induced vomiting may also complain about pain in the stomach or the intestines. Real damage to the liver and pancreas is entirely possible with this method of purging, just as your stomach, liver, intestines, heart, and brain were affected by the burden your alcoholic drinking placed on their normal functions.

When the urge to binge is rampant, the compulsive eater may very well practice another form of purging in secret, to get the taste of food without swallowing. He or she does this by simply chewing the food to get the flavor, and therefore the gratification, and then spitting it out so as not to put on more weight.

Purging food by using laxatives obviously eliminates the irritation to the lining of the esophagus and the mouth and does not cause tooth decay. But instead of all of that, laxatives damage the intestines and disrupt the body's electrolyte balance as much as vomiting.

Maybe worse, once the body gets used to having laxatives and indeed becomes dependent on them, muscles that were designed to move food through the intestines become lazy and no longer work. So the person not only becomes dependent on a destructive behavior pattern, he or she also becomes dependent on a new set of chemicals (laxatives) to help control body processes. And, as one might expect from addictive behavior, once the body develops a tolerance for a certain amount of laxatives, increasingly large doses are required to obtain the same results.

Remember, the compulsive eater is typically a perfectionist, which is part of his or her downfall in the first place. He or she sets what appear to be reasonable goals for behavior and appearance, but when he or she gets close to reaching those goals, the standards are raised, thus eliminating any possibility of real fulfillment.

Overeaters, like alcoholics, frequently have very low self-esteem; it was, after all, the alcohol that allowed them to feel good about themselves. These low "self-esteemers" feel they are not even worthy of living sometimes, much less being cared about. Their guilt feelings about their abnormal eating behaviors fuel their feelings of general inadequacy and of being unable to cope.

Compulsive eaters who are also recovering alcoholics are usually of normal weight, or within 10 to 15 pounds of that figure. Nevertheless, they may continue to feed "that little kid" inside them and then, fraught with guilt, "punish that kid" by self-induced vomiting or abusing laxatives.

At the opposite extreme from the "binging-then-purging" syndrome is a disorder we call anorexia nervosa. Anorexia literally means "not having an appetite." In the beginning, this syndrome tends to be more psychological than physical.

People suffering from this disorder frequently start off by losing an appropriate amount of weight. They will get many compliments on their appearance and persistence. This, of course, feeds "that little kid" a good dose of self-esteem. Well, the person about to become anorexic thrives on that sort of thing and so continues to lose weight, regardless of what is healthy. Body image becomes distorted and strange things happen. The obviously and excessively thin person begins to think of himself or herself as fat. Female patients will say "I'll gain weight if you'll tell me how to put the fat on my breasts—but my thighs are too big!" Sounds reasonable enough, except that the patient speaking has broomsticks for arms and legs and absolutely no chance of having fat thighs.

The idea here is to have the figure of a 15-year-old when the calendar clearly shows you're 40. It is a fact of life that women's bodies will not maintain their adolescent shape, especially not after the stressful changes of pregnancy and lactation.

The anorexic falls into the trap of continuing to lose weight even though his or her original goal was reached long ago. Compulsive thinking about food becomes more obvious. Food is the enemy to be controlled, just as she controls her body.

Each meal is planned in great detail. The anorexic is preoccupied with food. The fine touch of gourmet cooking is often noticeable in the meals an anorexic will prepare for others. Of course, he or she will eat like a bird or not at all! Anorexics become real pros at cutting an apple into, say, 17 pieces and eating them with a fork. It looks like a lot of eating is going on there, but it isn't.

Listening to an anorexic recite the calorie content of every food is like listening to an alcoholic recite the proper number of drinks that he or she can consume without getting "out of control." When confronted, anorexic patients strongly deny that anything is wrong with them and will become enraged at the suggestion that they "might need help." Sound familiar?

Active alcoholics may not intentionally set out to starve themselves as anorexics do, yet every time they skip meals in order to continue drinking, they are performing the same damaging ritual.

Not content with just one disorder, people will often alternate between the "binge-purge" and the anorexic syndromes. The end result of all this usually turns out to be a normal weight and compulsive and very secretive behavior that perpetuates low self-esteem.

So, the next time you are on the road to your second piece of pie or you find the ice cream dish starting to look more like a model of Mount Everest, pull in the reigns and recognize that, as an alcoholic in recovery, you have successfully given up the booze, but you may not have yet broken free of the behaviors that are leading you from one addiction to another.

CAFFEINE, NICOTINE, AND THOU

Admit it. You already knew the bad news, didn't you?

Somewhere in your mind was lurking the fact that alcohol *and* caffeine *and* nicotine are all bad for you. Without going into all the psychological factors of addiction, we are simply going to tell you what havoc caffeine and nicotine wreak on your body from a nutritional standpoint.

Whether or not you stop smoking and give up or cut down on your coffee drinking is, of course, a personal choice. When you entered recovery, you realized that alcoholism, being fatal if untreated, was getting the best of you, and you made the decision to stop drinking and start the sobriety process. Your body is getting better for it, not to mention your judgment and performance in all areas of your life.

With all three substances—alcohol, caffeine, and nicotine—the body's ability to utilize vitamins A and C, the B complex, zinc, calcium, and magnesium is undermined. With any one of them there is the possibility of developing nutritional deficiencies or perhaps imbalances that can lead to physical symptoms.

Ulcers are a clear and present danger from the abuse of all three of these substances. The blood sugar suffers also. The blood sugar levels get on a sort of roller coaster when any one substance is being used, but the effect is heightened by the use of more than one. In fact, if you use these substances in combination, which is highly likely, you more than double the negative impact.

We're certain that you may have already been discouraged from tackling more than one addiction at a time. You need to concentrate on your recovery from alcoholism. When your sobriety is well established and you are feeling secure with your new lifestyle, then is a good time to look at these other addictions—nicotine and caffeine.

It's a fact of life that persons who abuse one of these substances are more likely to abuse one or more of the others. All three substances are physically and psychologically addicting, so it's easy to justify what you have done over the years, smoking with your booze and with your coffee, or any combination of the three.

During your recovery process, it's highly likely that you have increased your use of caffeine and nicotine, relying on them as an emotional crutch, now that your "best friend" alcohol is out of the picture.

Caffeine

Caffeine and related substances, called xanthines, act as stimulants to both the central nervous system and the heart. Caffeine also stimulates gastric secretions, acts as a smooth-muscle relaxant, increases the need to urinate, and causes enough stresslike reactions in the body to raise the blood sugar (glucose) and free up fatty acids, which also circulate in the blood.

You get your peak blood-level "high" from caffeine within about an hour. Caffeine is absorbed directly and rather rapidly from the gastrointestinal tract, and you become aware of its effects equally rapidly.

Five ounces of coffee produce 60 to 180 milligrams of caffeine. On a dosage of, say, 50 to 200 milligrams, you experience increased alertness and less drowsiness. You're inclined to feel less bored and tired, and your attention is a lot sharper. You feel "on the ball" and "ready to hit it."

Those all appear to be positive effects of caffeine. But the other side of the coin shows that these same doses produce a situation in which difficult tasks may become more difficult to execute. Complex behavior patterns may become disrupted. However, tasks which you are used to performing and which you do with ease will be performed smoothly and efficiently.

If there are beneficial effects to caffeine, they are usually achieved with an intake of 250 to 300 milligrams, or one to three cups of coffee daily. If that's what you drink, and you're accustomed to it, then this amount appears to have little or no effect on nutritional health. When you start getting to larger amounts, the potential for causing major health problems increases. Why? Because of the caffeine's effects on the heart, stomach, kidneys, and nerves. You need to give serious consideration, even in recovery, to limiting the amount of coffee you drink. It's not uncommon to see recovering alcoholics put away 30 to 50 cups of coffee a day, using this substance in the same addictive fashion they were using alcohol. High doses of caffeine create a medical condition known as caffeinism. The symptoms are often indistinguishable from symptoms we would associate with anxiety, hence anxiety disorders.

Caffeinism shows up as nervousness, irritability, tremors, muscle spasms or twitching, insomnia, and rapid breathing. Add to the list of complaints disturbances of sight, hearing, and touch; irregular heartbeat; flushing; excessive urination; and last, but definitely not least, irritations of the stomach and intestine.

People are often surprised to find that they have raised their caffeine intake up to 2,000 milligrams or more a day. But they get caffeine from many sources, not just coffee. We've included a chart to help you define your own caffeine-milligram intake. Consider this: an intake within a fairly short period of time of 100 or more milligrams can be toxic for the person who has a low caffeine tolerance level. Just 900 milligrams causes an increase in specialized liver enzymes that are needed for detoxification. Five hundred milligrams increases your metabolic rate, that is, the rate at which your body uses calories, by 10 to 25 percent.

Let's look deeper into your system and find the other effects of caffeine on the body. Starting down in your stomach, caffeine causes increased secretion of acid, which in turn might be enough to cause an ulcer. Acid secretion is higher and lasts for longer periods of time in the person who already has an ulcer, of course. The same applies to gastric irritation in the ulcerated person.

Some medical researchers have reported that instant and decaffeinated coffee are even more potent stimulants of acid than regular coffee or even pure caffeine. Blood pressure is affected by caffeine also. Caffeine increases the force of the contractions in the heart, resulting in increased blood flow and higher blood pressure. But this effect is somewhat masked by another effect of caffeine. The use of caffeine decreases heart rate.

An irregular heartbeat might be detected in the caffeine user, or there may be no obvious symptoms for a long period of time. Blood vessels in the body become dilated by caffeine, but the ones in the brain are constricted. This constriction can happen with as little as 500 milligrams of caffeine. Therefore, blood flow to the brain diminishes, while blood flow to the rest of the body increases.

Medical specialists have not yet established a direct link between coronary heart disease and caffeine intake, but we do know that caffeine consumption affects cholesterol. How? As caffeine consumption increases, so do cholesterol levels. It certainly won't do you any harm to keep your caffeine consumption at low or moderate levels, instead of waiting for some research team to make the connection.

We all know that drinking a lot of coffee increases the need to urinate. Well, caffeine is a diuretic, just like alcohol, and so it also washes away a lot of good things we need, such as those important water-soluble vitamins C and B complex, along with all minerals, especially zinc and magnesium.

If you already have a marginal intake of these nutrients, then the impact of your daily consumption of caffeine will need to be carefully considered. Again, for the well-nourished person, drinking one or two cups of coffee a day makes very little difference. We're not talking about the two-cup-a-day coffee drinker, but about the caffeine abuser.

Caffeine is an addicting substance, and you can experience definite withdrawal symptoms and cravings for it. It's also an "upper," unlike alcohol and nicotine, which are "downers." You raise your blood sugar levels when you use caffeine; adding sugar to your coffee just makes things worse. If you also smoke, then you are sending double messages to your body and your blood sugar levels will keep going up and down like some crazy elevator.

If you have suffered liver damage or have liver disease, then the caffeine you consume is processed and eliminated much more slowly then in the average person. Instead of breaking down the caffeine and eliminating it within a few hours, your body might retain it for a day or longer. The longer you continue to consume caffeine, the more you build up for your body to process.

Withdrawal symptoms familiar to all of you who have tried breaking your coffee habits are severe headaches lasting as long as two weeks, vomiting, nausea, and general crankiness. Withdrawal can be so severe that in one case a person admitted himself to the emergency room of a local hospital, certain that he was suffering a stroke.

Gradually reducing the amount of caffeine consumed is probably an easier way to eliminate caffeine from your diet than going "cold turkey." In recovery, you will be better off using decaffeinated coffee to decrease the impact of caffeine on your blood sugar levels. When you control these levels, you are helping to control the stress that the blood sugar fluctuations cause. Steam-decaffeinated coffee is a better choice than the products that use chemicals to remove the caffeine from the coffee beans.

Common Sources of Caffeine

Coffee (5 ounces)

Brewed, drip method	60–180 mg.
Brewed, percolator	40–170 mg.
Instant	30–120 mg.
Decaffeinated, brewed	2–5 mg.
Decaffeinated, instant	1–5 mg.

Tea (5 ounces)

Brewed, major U.S. brands	20–90 mg.
Brewed, imported	25–110 mg.
Instant	25–50 mg.
Iced (12 ounces)	67–76 mg.

Chocolate

Cocoa (5 ounces)	2–20 mg.
Chocolate milk (8 ounces)	2–7 mg.
Milk chocolate (1 ounce)	1–15 mg.
Semisweet chocolate (1 ounce)	5–35 mg.
Chocolate candy bar, small	25 mg.

Soft drinks (12 ounces)	30–60 mg.

Pain medications

Excedrin (standard dose)	60–130 mg.

Stimulants

No Doz (standard dose)	100–200 mg.
Weight-control medications	200–280 mg.
Cold medications	30 mg.

Note: Caffeine is also present in coffee-flavored desserts such as mocha ice cream, cake, or pie.

Sources: Food and Drug Administration; *FDA Consumer*, March 1984; *Tufts University Nutrition Newsletter*, April 1984.

Nicotine

This substance interferes with the absorption of calcium and is often a primary factor in the development of adult bone loss, called osteoporosis. Nicotine interferes with the absorption of other minerals, causing imbalances that could eventually produce deficiency syndromes in persons with poor nutrition. That's just for openers.

Smoke and nicotine irritate the mucous membranes of both the lungs and the gastrointestinal tract. This irritation of the lining of the stomach increases the risk of ulcers and all the complications resulting from that little problem.

Increased cholesterol and triglyceride levels have been definitely linked to nicotine, and you are all aware of the risk of coronary heart disease associated with fatty deposits in the blood vessels. These deposits increase with nicotine use. Should we mention higher blood pressure caused by constriction of blood vessels? How about the extra strain nicotine places on your heart by increasing cholesterol deposits? There's very little good to say about the use of nicotine.

Stress accompanies the use of nicotine. Why? Because a stresslike reaction occurs when the nicotine stimulates the adrenal glands in your body, thus raising blood sugar levels (remember?). Now we get fluctuating blood sugar levels and the hypoglycemia-like reactions experienced by many recovering persons.

More news about nicotine. One cigarette suppresses your appetite for 15 to 60 minutes, so smokers frequently smoke instead of eating, or they delay their intake of food. Not good! The suppression of appetite occurs as a result of three factors: namely, the increase in blood sugar levels, the deadening of the taste buds, and the inhibiting of stomach contractions. As you have already been told, skipping meals reduces your caloric intake and thus places you, the smoker, at a possible nutritional risk. The use of nicotine also increases the metabolic rate, so smokers eat more and gain less weight, a trick they often rely on to justify the continued use of nicotine.

Finally, nicotine acts as a body stimulant. When this stimulant effect wears off, you feel more relaxed. Nicotine stimulates the flow of adrenaline, increases the heart rate, and the strength of heart contractions. All of that, of course, constricts blood vessels, causing higher blood pressure. Cholesterol and free fatty acids are generally higher in smokers. Nicotine interferes with red blood cells, which transport oxygen throughout the body, and therefore with cell metabolism as well.

Nicotine causes starvation at a cellular level, and its impact may not be seen for years. Nicotine interferes with your body's ability to use vitamins C, B_{12}, and B_6. It depletes vital magnesium, calcium, and phosphorus, and interferes with your body's ability to process and utilize carbohydrates and protein.

Well, it's up to you. Recovering from one fatal disease is hard enough. To court disaster by abusing a different drug just doesn't make sense. The choice is yours, but the conclusion should be shouting at you loud and clear.

GROWING A SWEET TOOTH?

Americans rely on sugar or other sweeteners in their diets. Some experts believe that sugar affects the mental functions, as well as the mood, of an individual. Like any drug, sugar can be addicting; many people cannot live without it. Are you one of them?

Some vitamins produce significant physiological and psychological changes, even when they are taken in minute quantities. Does this make them drugs also? Well, let's look at the bottom line here. The determination should be whether or not the substance—sugar, vitamin, or drug—is used for the purpose of altering mood or body sensations. If a person cannot go for a period of time without using the substance, then it is said to be addicting.

You've seen the "sugar addict." This is the person who might consume one candy bar, two or three pieces of peanut brittle, a couple of chocolate chip cookies, all within a ten-minute period of waiting for his bus.

Sugar is not a poison, but a source of carbohydrate calories. It contributes no vitamins, minerals, fiber, protein, or other substance of redeeming value to the body's nutritional requirements.

Did you know that the average American will consume 120 pounds or more of refined sweetener each year? Consider this: 70 to 80 percent of the sugar consumed comes from foods prepared outside the home. Americans like the taste of sugar. The average fast-food hamburger, for example, contains approximately 9 teaspoons of sugar! How does this affect you, particularly if you are in the recovery process?

Recovering persons use sugar to help them get through the difficult period of withdrawal from alcohol and to deal with fluctuations in their blood-sugar levels, which are part of that recovery process. In the early stages of recovery, the use of high-sugar foods (ice cream and lemonade are typical) seems to be appropriate.

But used in copious amounts as a mood-altering substance, sugar becomes addicting. Sugar, however, is a depressant and, consumed in large amounts, it affects the opiate receptor sites in the central nervous system. Here's how this works. As the sedative, or relaxing, effects of sugar wear off, you may experience agitation or a feeling of being "hyper." This is a rebound reaction that starts that old roller coaster of feeling first "up," then "down," just like the cross-use between alcohol, caffeine, and nicotine. In fact sugar, when combined with caffeine, seems to have a more addicting effect.

Using large amounts of coffee loaded with sugar is essentially the same as combining an upper and a downer.

By the way, the practice of combining substances whose effects oppose each other appears to be common among recovering persons.

So what's our "beef" with the use of sugar? Our primary concern is with the amount consumed and its possible impact on your health and hence your full recovery from the disease of alcoholism. If the sugar you use replaces foods that provide essential nutrients, then the possibility of malnutrition arises.

In order for your body to process sugar so that it can be used for energy, B-complex vitamins, zinc, magnesium, and other trace minerals must be present. But sugar provides none of these, only calories. Sure, you can take a "one-a-day" vitamin to make up for the good stuff you are missing when you get most of your calories from sugar and fat, but what about the other health problems that stem from an excessive consumption of sugar?

For example, what about tooth decay and periodontal disease? Do you really want to run the risk of colon cancer due to inadequate fiber intake? How about coronary heart disease due to high fat intake? There is always, of course, the possibility that you will become addicted to sugar (you are at high risk for addiction anyhow) and will then need to be treated for that substance abuse, just as for the alcohol.

Some of the experts in the field of stress management and behavioral science feel that sugar increases the body's stress load and adrenaline reactions. We have seen patients with many allergies and have observed that a high sugar intake seems to affect the immune system. It does so to the point that there is an increased susceptibility to disease organisms and very possibly to allergens.

But the sugar junkie is a lot like the alcoholic who has

convinced himself or herself that the use of the substance "doesn't really hurt." "Sugar is a food, and so it's
natural," says the afflicted person. If a decision to use
only "natural foods" has been made, then the deception
is even greater. The sweeteners that are used in a
"natural foods" diet may include honey, date sugar,
molasses, and concentrated fruit juice, instead of sugar.
This would be done, of course, in the false belief that
these sweeteners are less harmful. No matter what the
source of sweetener, however, excessive amounts are
detrimental to health and to the recovery process.

Just like alcoholics, persons who are addicted to
sugar are preoccupied with it. They make elaborate
plans for their "sugar fixes," frequently consuming
these foods with great ritual or under specific circumstances. The sugar addict will see to it that he or she
gets regular fixes during the day, usually in the form of
doughnuts, cookies, candies, or soda. This is in addition
to the regular foods he or she consumes, which will also
be high in sugar. And, also like the alcoholic, once this
sugar junkie starts eating the sugar, he or she can't stop
until a certain degree of satiation is reached—it's just
like the alcoholic who doesn't take one or two drinks,
but drinks to get drunk.

The compulsion to eat sugar is constant. When sugar
is not available, the person addicted to it might feel
depressed or agitated because something is missing.
There is no question that withdrawal from sugar can be
as painful as withdrawal from alcohol. It has been
described by those who have undergone both as
"worse."

With sugar substitutes, you can have the sweetness of
sugar without the calories and the possible negative
effects of sugar. However, there is a big difference
between sugar and sugar substitutes, in addition to the
difference in calorie content. A non-nutritive sweetener
only tastes sweet and does not satisfy appetite. This
might account for the fact that some persons consume
more high-fat foods when they use sugar substitutes.

They do this convinced that, having "saved calories" with the non-nutritive sweetener, they can make up the difference elsewhere. But some non-nutritive sweeteners actually increase the appetite and therefore add to the problem rather than reduce it. There are questions of safety: Do these chemicals cause cancer? Are there are other health problems associated with these sweeteners? Research is still being done to find answers.

The primary sugar substitutes on the market today are saccharine, aspartame, and substances called polyols, such as manitol, sorbitol, and xylitol. These polyols are sweet-tasting alcohols that have 2 calories per gram as opposed to the 4 calories per gram found in sugar. They taste a lot sweeter than sugar, so very small amounts can be used to achieve the same flavor. They are used primarily in candy and gum, where they have the extra advantage of not causing tooth decay.

Saccharine has been with us since the beginning of the twentieth century. It is 300 times sweeter than sugar, so minute amounts can be used to produce the desired degree of sweetness. Every so often (fairly regularly, it seems), questions arise as to the safety of saccharine. Warning labels are now required to indicate that the use of this product may cause cancer. At one time, it was proposed that saccharine be taken off the market, but the outraged American public quickly vetoed the idea. So it remains.

The newest sugar substitute is aspartame. You see it regularly in diet or sugar-free products that list NutraSweet among their ingredients. This is a brand name for aspartame. When you buy packets of this sugar substitute for home use, you will find it marketed under the trade name Equal. Aspartame has 4 calories per gram, but it is 180 times sweeter than sugar. Only very small amounts are needed to provide a sweetened taste. Aspartame is composed of two amino acids, phenylalanine and aspartic acid, which occur normally in food.

Aspartame appears to be the safest non-nutritive sweetener developed so far; the majority of the questions it has raised concern individual consumption of and sensitivity to the product. Some cases of adverse reaction have been reported and are under investigation, but only a relatively small percentage of consumers have reported problems.

Aspartame is everywhere—in soft drinks, medications, you name it. This raises the possibility of overloading the body with two amino acids and causing nutritional imbalances. Aspartame has been proven to increase feelings of hunger and decrease feelings of fullness within an hour of eating foods that contain it. The theory has been advanced that aspartame may disrupt the appetite control center of the brain and cause the person using it to eat more rather than less.

Alcoholics in recovery have been known to strike up a great friendship with aspartame, in what appears to be a fairly addictive pattern. Patients have reported using from 14 to 18 cans of diet soda a day. Another case reviewed found a recovering person using 50 packets of aspartame *per day* in hot water with lemon juice or instant coffee. The need in both cases appeared to be for the aspartame, as opposed to the caffeine found in the soda or instant coffee. Other recovering persons reported feeling dependent on aspartame and experienced withdrawal symptoms when giving it up. They also said they just "didn't feel well" if they didn't have aspartame. Based on the present knowledge of the possible effects of amino acid imbalances on the brain, addiction or dependency on aspartame certainly seems possible, but has not been proven.

The recovering person is advised to use sugar substitutes in moderation. You are better off learning the real flavors of foods without tampering with their taste. Learn to prefer foods with very little or no sweetener of any kind added. Learn to really enjoy the taste, aroma, and full-bodied flavor that nature provides us in so many fruits and vegetables. You will be better off nutritionally and spiritually.

If you feel you have been overusing sugar and sugar

substitutes, consider the possibility that you (yes, *you*) may be trading one addiction, alcohol, for another, sugar. Isn't dealing with *one* addiction just about enough? Life can be sweet for you on a natural basis. Go for it!

TO SUPPLEMENT
OR NOT TO SUPPLEMENT

As recently as November 1986, a report came out of the Soviet Union that the Soviets were using fasting successfully in treating alcoholism. In the same month, U.S. researchers reported on a new experimental drug, being tested on laboratory rats, that apparently sobered the animals within 3 minutes of being injected. The usual warnings were sounded that this treatment was "highly experimental" and "not necessarily a cure" for alcoholism.

At the same time, we here in the United States have been overtaken with all kinds of nutritional therapies, which have in themselves become thriving businesses. There are all kinds of books and articles describing miraculous cures and suggesting that the craving for alcohol will be almost instantaneously relieved if a certain diet is followed or a certain supplement is used.

There are many self-proclaimed nutritional experts out there preaching similar messages on radio, television, and in the print media. The bottom line with most of these, we have found, is the necessity of purchasing a specific product or specially packaged line of goods.

When surveys are taken among the public, there is evidence of widespread confusion about nutritional supplements, as well as a ready supply of misinformation. We do know that approximately 40 percent of the American public use nutritional supplements daily and that the use of vitamin supplements is a fact of life for most people. The question is not whether one should take the supplements, but rather which ones and what amounts to take.

Now, if you have been following this book carefully
and adhering to our advice about eating a variety of
foods from the four basic food groups every day, you
won't normally need any vitamin or mineral supplements. Not only would they be unnecessary, but they
might actually increase stress levels by causing an
overdose to which your body would have to adapt.

Because you became dependent on alcohol in the
past, in recovery you want to avoid building another
dependency, even on vitamin and mineral supplements.
You want to be self-sufficient, to be as healthy as
possible, and not to depend on anything. That's natural
enough, but in attaining that self-sufficiency you may
have put your nutritional needs at the very bottom of
your list.

Face it, honestly! When you were drinking, the
number one priority was drinking, and you probably
didn't even bother with eating regularly. Maybe you
took vitamins, particularly if you believed that doing so
would decrease the probability of liver damage. Oh,
you might have eaten regularly enough if you had had
someone preparing your meals or if you had had
sufficient means to eat in restaurants all the time, but
even then you would have skipped meals. You could get
drunker faster if you skipped meals altogether.

You know, like all alcoholics, that if there was ever a
choice between buying food and alcohol, the booze
won, hands down. The chances are pretty good that
when you did choose food, it was not for its nutritional
value but more for its ease of preparation or consumption. However, as we have discussed earlier in this book,
when you were using the alcohol, you were depleting
your nutritional reserves. You were also preventing the
absorption and utilization of what vitamins and minerals you did manage to get into your diet.

Since your body is marvelously adaptable, you probably didn't present clinical symptoms of nutritional
deficiencies when you entered recovery. But even if
there were no overt signs of a nutritional deficiency, you

probably had some marginal deficiencies that remained. The first sign of such a deficiency is psychological and shows up as "just not feeling well."

Substance abuse counselors have a bona fide concern about the possibility that their patients, including you, might trade dependency on one substance (alcohol) for another (supplements). Why? Because various vitamins can produce a sense of well-being. Since vitamins and minerals come from food and are therefore natural, they cannot hurt and might even help the recovery process. You should remind yourself, however, that you can get too much of a good thing. The primary goal of your recovery is to learn to care for yourself without depending on extraneous substances. In reality, though, a moderate use of nutritional supplements seems to help the recovery process for most people.

So the obvious question arises: namely, what supplements are appropriate, when should they be taken, and for how long? For the recovering person, use this table of supplements as your guide.

DAILY SUPPLEMENTS

Vitamin B_1	1.5–5 mg
Vitamin B_2	1.7–5 mg
Niacin	15–50 mg
Vitamin B_6	2–6 mg
Vitamin B_{12}	3–10 mcg
Folate	400–800 mcg
Vitamin C	100–500 mg (for smokers)
Zinc	15–30 mg
Magnesium	350–500 mg

A one-a-day multivitamin would provide these nutrients plus 5,000 IU (International Units) of vitamin A, 200 to 400 IU of vitamin D, and 15 to 30 IU of vitamin E.

Persons who can't or *won't* eat dairy foods daily need calcium supplements. One serving of a dairy food contains 300 milligrams of calcium. The recommended amounts are 800 to 1,000 milligrams for men, and 1,000 to 1,500 milligrams for women.

In the early stages of your recovery, and probably well into the first year, even if you eat well, it is advisable for you to take supplements of the B vitamins, vitamin C, and zinc. We make this recommendation on the assumption that you are eating a varied diet from the four basic food groups, including vitamin D–fortified milk, raw fruits and vegetables, along with adequate amounts of meat, fish, poultry, eggs, and whole grains to meet your protein and carbohydrate needs.

Your emphasis should be on the water-soluble nutrients that are most affected by alcohol. These are the ones that you are likely to be deficient in and the ones most needed to assist you in recovering.

Keep in mind that megadoses of vitamins and minerals are not advised unless recommended by a physician. Overdoses can occur. They can cause additional damage or can slow recovery rather than help it. As a general rule, any dose that is three times the RDA (Recommended Daily Allowance) is not advised. Your physician should be the one to decide if higher doses are warranted.

Taking small amounts of B-complex vitamins four to six times a day has been helpful in overcoming a difficult stage of recovery called the "dry drunk." We recommend breaking low-potency B vitamins into quarter pieces and taking one of the pieces every two to three hours. You may find that shopping for these low-potency vitamins in this era of megadoses is an interesting experience. You'll probably find yourself looking at lots of generic brands or those brands stashed away on the bottom shelves of your market or pharmacy. Health-food store clerks might give you a lively argument about why you should use the megadoses, but stick to your guns.

These recommendations are intended to help you meet your daily needs without becoming dependent on supplements or laboring under the illusion that vitamin and mineral supplements are the answer to all your problems.

Your primary source of nutrients should always be food. Those foods that have been fortified to the point that they are nothing but vitamin pills disguised as breakfast cereals or protein drinks or bread aren't going to do a whole lot for you.

What you need here is commitment. You have to be willing to use foods that are processed as little as possible. You have to be willing and able to avoid prepared foods 80 to 90 percent of the time. If you do this, then the need for supplements of any kind is drastically reduced, since you will be getting the nutrients you need from your diet.

In the first stages of recovery, you will need the help provided by appropriate supplementation with vitamins and minerals. The symptoms of nutritional imbalances that may show up, particularly in your first year of recovery, may make it necessary for you to use these supplements for a longer period of time. The physician who is monitoring your recovery program is the best judge of this. Supplements are not *the* answer to complete and successful recovery. They, like all the other tools that are provided to you, are to be considered carefully and used wisely.

9
Table for One?

Have you ever had to face the embarrassment of asking, "Table for one, please"? If you are a recovering person, you haven't had much practice in doing this, because it's pretty likely that you didn't eat properly at all, whether you were alone or with dozens of people.

In this chapter we are going to address the recovering alcoholic who may live alone, or the recovering person who has discovered the joy of cooking (and eating) for the first time. We will talk about shopping wisely, cooking for yourself, eating alone, and not putting yourself down because of it. Singles and single parents with teenagers in the home have more in common than one might imagine, since mealtimes for single parents may very well be as solitary as if there weren't other people in the house.

The teen "eating machines" get their food pretty much on the run, leaving you perhaps to fend for yourself. Alcoholics, as a general class of people, don't do too well being alone to start with. This is one of the dynamics that makes the booze bottle such a "good and trusted friend." There's not a lot of reason to suppose that the recovering person will feel any better if he or she is alone. What's important, though, is to treat yourself as well as you can, whether you are by yourself or not.

SHOPPING FOR ONE

We'll begin with the hard part, and that's shopping for one. We know that people who live alone, or at least don't have anyone with whom to share meals, tend to whip their shopping carts right past the fresh vegetables at the market. Their rationale is they can't possibly use them up before they spoil, so they don't buy them in the first place. This problem is easily solved. Ask the produce clerk to cut vegetables such as cabbage and cauliflower, so that smaller amounts can be purchased. He'll be glad to accommodate you and you can buy just what you can use in a week's time.

You really pay for broccoli by the pound and not by the bunch, so it's no big deal to break up those bunches that have been conveniently tied and take one or two stalks instead of five, six, or seven in the bunch. Green peppers and onions can be frozen just the way they are; no blanching is necessary. Use them straight out of the freezer in cooking or partially thawed in your salad.

Canned fruits and vegetables are more expensive in the smaller cans, but in the long run they make less waste and therefore save you money. Or you can pick up some of those plastic freezer containers, use the larger cans of fruit, separate them into smaller portions, and freeze or refrigerate the excess. Your best bet is to purchase frozen fruits and vegetables that come in the bags, so that you can prepare only the amount needed.

With all the rush to the salad bars these days (sure beats the booze bars!), many singles find it helpful to purchase precut vegetables at the bar, take them home,

and cook them or use them in their own salads with a
prepared meal. Don't be afraid to ask the butcher to cut
smaller portions of meat or cheese for you. If you take
the time, you can purchase a larger cut of meat, prepare
the whole cut, and cut and freeze the portions. Some
grocers will even sell you half loaves of bread. But if
this service isn't available, go ahead and buy your
bread, divide it, and freeze what you won't be using immediately.

When you shop, you need to be aware that highly
processed imitation foods do not have the same nutrient values as natural foods. The profit margin on
processed imitation foods is high, and a lot of advertising dollars are spent to make sure that you the consumer are aware of them.

Basic foods are carried, believe it or not, as a necessity. The processed foods provide the bulk of sales to
consumers and receive the greatest amount of display
space. Items that you use on a daily basis are generally
to be found in the back of the store, with the "come-on"
items brightly and attractively displayed to grab you
when you first enter.

As you are undoubtedly aware, supermarkets are laid
out to serve the neighborhoods in which they are
located. A store in an area with lots of children is going
to have tons of candy display space, snack counters, and
a general look of "quick foods" to it. If your store is
located in an area that caters primarily to busy professionals, for whom the quick lunch or dinner is important, then you will probably find the deli section near
the front of the store. And so on.

The point is, you will have to keep in mind the four
basic food groups. Locate them in your store and make
them the first places you visit, avoiding the impulse
items.

Once you realize that reaching the four basic food
groups means having to pass the processed and prepared foods, you can be on the alert. Think about it. To

get to the fresh vegetables, fruit, milk, poultry, meat, and fish, you probably have to head for the rear of the supermarket. Boy, will you pass a lot of other items on your way there!

Living alone creates a temptation to live primarily on convenience foods such as pizza, frozen dinners, and canned spaghetti and ravioli. Not only do these foods hit you pretty hard in the pocketbook, but they are of questionable nutritional value as well. What's the reason for this? Well, you can't assume that the companies preparing these foods use the same types of ingredients that you would choose if you were preparing them from scratch. After all, the primary goal of the food supplier is to make a profit. So it's safe to suppose that the "substitution rule" is at work. This is the rule that says, "If you can substitute a cheaper (and perhaps less nutritious) ingredient for the one usually found in this food, then do it."

You may very well find items such as tomatoes, cheese, fruit, butter, cream, and even meat replaced under the "substitution rule" with texturized starch, modified soy protein, or torula yeast.

"Wait a minute!" you cry. "How can that tomato paste be phony?" Simple. When added to the right juice, such as apple or tomato, texturized starch can appear to be tomato paste. It can also be made to look like fruit or cream fillings. "Well, they can't do that with meat!" comes your indignant challenge. "Yes, they can!" is the reply. Soy protein and torula yeast can be made into substances that resemble meat and cheese. Oh, they have some nutritional value alright, but not nearly the same value as the foods they replace.

Adding extra water or sugar can alter the nutrient density in convenience foods also. They may look the same as the foods you would prepare at home, yet have very different nutritional value. Regulations on food labels require that a food that is labeled "natural" contain 10 percent natural ingredients. That leaves a lot of room for the food producers to dilute the real food with ingredients of little or no food value.

Just look at all the imitation foods on the shelves these days. Consumers are generally under the impression that the nutrient value of these imitations is the same as that of the real things. Not so. Fruit drinks are colored and flavored sugar water with vitamin C added perhaps. But that's where the resemblance to the real thing stops. The other nutrients besides vitamin C that are found in real fruit—the vitamin A, potassium, and other trace minerals—are absent from the fake product.

Cream substitutes are a mixture of coconut oil, corn sweetener, and flavoring, and all you get out of that is more calories. Frozen and canned puddings contain little or no milk and thus are nothing more than a source of calories. Read labels carefully and take the information on those labels literally. Frequently, food labels are worded in such a way that we read information into them and assume a lot more than is actually stated. Also, just because a product is labeled "natural" doesn't necessarily mean it's all natural. It must contain only 10 percent natural ingredients to earn the "natural" label.

Packages are designed in nice earth tones of browns, yellows, and greens to help move products into your grocery cart. Don't be taken in by packaging. When you're looking at the labels on foods, the nutritional information will give you facts about calories, carbohydrates, protein, and fat levels. In addition, there will be a statement about the percentage of the RDA (recommended daily allowance) of specific nutrients.

The more you read and learn about package information, the greater your inclination will be to decrease the amount of processed foods you buy and to turn more toward fresh or minimally processed foods.

What we are leading up to is the big pitch to get you to prepare at least some of your own food at home. It's not as hard as it may seem.

Planning ahead and keeping foods with high nutrient value in stock will help simplify things. What are the high-nutrient foods that will also keep well?

Try carrots, celery, green pepper, cabbage, broccoli, cauliflower, apples, and oranges. These foods will keep well in your refrigerator for up to two weeks without spoiling or losing significant amounts of nutrients.

If you have a hard time keeping milk, then try yogurt. It will last longer and it can be used very satisfactorily on your cereal. Add some fruit and you've got good eating. Get the milk you want when you eat out.

Keep powdered milk in your pantry. It can be added to sauces and homemade quick breads such as biscuits, pancakes, or muffins. Put it in with scrambled eggs or soup and give yourself extra calcium. Powdered milk has a long shelf life, so it's a good investment.

No decent larder is complete without whole-grain cereals such as Grape-Nuts or Shredded Wheat. These are great cereals for your yogurt with fruit. They can be used as a snack as well as a breakfast meal. A high-protein breakfast can be obtained when you take only 5 to 10 minutes to prepare a hot grain cereal such as oatmeal. Add milk or yogurt, and you're all set.

Cheese is a good source of calcium, remember. It will keep longer than milk. When you choose low-fat cheese, you reduce your calorie intake, as well as the amount of saturated fats in your diet.

Buy yourself some small cans of garbanzo, pinto, and black beans. Stock some tuna, turkey, and salmon, and you've got the fixings for quick casseroles and sandwiches. If you want crackers for snacking or to go with your soups or salads, make them whole grain. They'll keep longer than bread, anyhow.

While we're on the subject of snacks, keep popcorn around. It's easy to fix, high in nutritive value, and, if you have an air popper, only 25 calories per cup. Dried fruits are great for snacks. They can also be added to hot whole-grain cereals for sweetness. These fruits are concentrated foods, so they are high in calories. You will want to monitor how much of them you eat.

Nuts, sunflower seeds, and pumpkin seeds make terrific snacks and keep well in the refrigerator. But there is a price to pay. They are high in calories, so use them sparingly.

Of course, you should keep a supply of frozen concentrated fruit juices fortified with vitamin C. They keep indefinitely, so stock up when special sales or promotions are going on. You'll save money that way.

Rice and pasta are two more foods for your pantry shelves. They keep for long periods of time and they cook up in a jiffy.

COOKING FOR ONE

Now, you may not relish the thought of spending hours in the kitchen. Funny, you didn't mind spending hours in a bar or cocktail lounge doing almost nothing except consuming a poison—alcohol.

Maybe the new you should take another look at the fun, relaxation, and sense of achievement that come with puttering around in the kitchen. Part of your new lifestyle of recovery involves taking some risks and being adventurous, so give this a try.

Part of your game plan when cooking for yourself is to use the right appliance. Use the ones that shorten preparation time or that can cook the meal while you do something else. Slow cookers, microwave ovens, and pressure cookers are often found (and used extensively) in the kitchens of folks who cook and dine alone. Blenders can shorten food preparation time when you cook for one, but your food processor will probably be more useful for meals for two or more.

When you get the hang of it, you'll be able to prepare quick breads from start to finish in 30 minutes. These really put some pizazz into a meal, whether it's for one or a dozen. Make them from whole-grain flour so you can increase your intake of fiber and B-complex vitamins. Whole-grain mixes can also be used for cookies and fruit breads, which will add variety to your life and make your solo meals more appealing.

Learn to prepare and package your own TV dinners. If you will set aside two or three hours twice a month to cook and then clean up your kitchen, you can package a lot of meals for later use. During this span of time you can prepare, say, four casseroles or enough main dishes to feed eight persons.

Get or save some of those plastic plates that you receive with your microwave dinners. Or you can use aluminum pie plates. It's simple: cook your meals, divide them in portions, and arrange them attractively on the individual plates and freeze them. When it's time for you to eat one of these dinners, supplement the main entree or casserole with a fresh vegetable or salad, add fresh fruit or dessert, and you have a very nutritious meal with lots of variety. If you want to cut down your preparation time even more, use your vegetables from the frozen food supply, taking just what you need from the bag and keeping the rest for another time.

When you try this system for a month or so, you will find the preparation time is well worth the effort, since you will be making enough meals of a wide and pleasant variety to last for quite a while.

Foods that can be prepared ahead of time include pasta dishes such as spaghetti or lasagna, pineapple chicken, meat loaf or salmon loaf, and Mexican dishes such as enchiladas, chili, and burritos.

You may have friends who live alone and eat alone, too. Well, you can plan and cook meals for each other and have the fun and satisfaction of feeding someone other than yourself—it's a real treat. Not only will you find yourself putting a little extra effort into your meal, but you will probably experiment a little more with new foods and food ideas as well.

When you are dining alone, make it special. You don't have to glue yourself in front of the TV. Set a special place for yourself, select some good music, and enjoy the meal you have prepared. It's a significant part of your recovery to be able to savor good food again and recognize its importance to your lifelong sobriety. Setting a special "table for one" helps you recognize your own importance. You are someone special and you need to give yourself some V.I.P. service.

You may have become so used to putting yourself down because of your alcoholism that even the simplest needs and pleasures (which others take for granted) have become real strangers in your life. So you develop a tendency to skip meals or have a dinner of popcorn only, rather than taking the time and making the effort to prepare something that smells good, looks good, and definitely tastes good. See if you don't begin to realize how important eating well is to your overall plan for recovery. You will also begin to realize how neglected this part of your life has become. You will gain a real sense of well-being and discovery when you become more involved in planning, preparing, and eating your own meals.

It's a new experience for you, not to be missed. So get going. Dress up your kitchen, dress up your life! A table for one awaits a very deserving person.

10
Eating Out: From Candlelight to Drive-Through

Do you sometimes feel you have more conversations with the speaker voice at your neighborhood "drive-through" than with members of your own family? Has your tendency to dine out increased over the last year? Are you spending more dollars and more time in restaurants these days? The answers, on the basis of national surveys, are all on the affirmative side.

Eating out is part of the American lifestyle. Statistics tell us that the average American eats out at least once a day. In the near future, we are being told, it will be common for us to be taking two meals a day away from home.

The preponderance of two-income families is partly responsible for this trend. With both adults working, it is difficult to rush home and fix a big meal for others. Throw in some teenagers with busy lifestyles of their own, and the American family just doesn't manage to sit down together for regular meals.

So how come they do it at a restaurant? Well, for one

thing, "going out to dinner" is still an occasion and members of a busy household will make room for it in their schedules. The fast-food craze that has swept America shows no signs of subsiding. Television advertising continues to show the fast-food restaurant as a place for family fun: a place where birthday parties are held or where a busy mom or dad takes "time out" for the little ones. These TV ads stress the fun and convenience of such places, not the nutritional values of the foods they serve, and understandably so. If you are on a special diet, if you are in recovery and trying hard to get on the right track nutritionally, these establishments should not be part of your life.

So many people conduct their business over meals that they consider meals a part of work time. Doing business also involves traveling. Eating meals on planes or in airport restaurants isn't a matter of convenience anymore, but rather a matter of necessity in the business world.

Carrying food along for such situations may make you seem "a little weird." The lack of refrigeration, proper preparation areas, etc., tend to make eating out the inevitable choice.

What you may not be aware of is the large variety of restaurants that are available: cafeterias, delis, "drive-throughs" with sit-down facilities, "candlelight and violin" restaurants, and more and more ethnic restaurants. Keep in mind that most ethnic restaurants usually serve the feast or holiday foods of the country they represent, not the fare of common folk. Look out for rich sauces, fried foods, and extra sugar and butter.

In any restaurant, it is important to be aware of calories, cholesterol, and sugar. Evaluate the menu carefully so that you can get the nutrients you need. Be picky about the foods you choose, rather than just accepting the "special of the day." There is a wide choice of dishes on most menus—choose what's best for you.

Deli counters in supermarkets are fast becoming indispensable to busy families. Food choices include not only fried foods and other high-fat items such as hotdogs, but also a vast array of salads, meats, and even low-sodium cheeses. The thing is, you need to ask for the low-fat items if you're serious about changing your nutritional life.

Deli eating has to do with convenience and not necessarily with nutrition. Vegetables, other than those in salads, are not prominent deli items. The emphasis is on the "quick bite to eat," and so you tend to pick up a lot of items of questionable value for their convenience.

Let's not overlook another institution of American food life that is becoming more visible with every passing month. That is the mobile food service affectionately called the "roach coach," or some other derogatory name. The mobile food service was originally designed to provide construction workers with a wide choice of foods including hot soups, sandwiches, and of course tons of desserts, candy bars, sodas, and coffee, coffee, coffee! But many office workers and executives now await the arrival of the "roach coach" for their midday break or lunch needs. Some of the more enterprising of these businesses will bring meals right into the hallways of the most modern offices, all to save you the trouble of leaving your desk to eat.

Chain restaurants that don't provide drive-through services offer standardized menus with some variations to suit the season or the locale. These places employ equipment similar to that of the drive-through operations, allowing for relatively quick sit-down service.

Unless you choose to pay more to eat in a restaurant that cooks everything from scratch and has a varied menu, you will find your diet limited by the choices offered. After all, a primary concern of eating establishments is to keep food costs down and profits high, and limiting their menus is one important way to accomplish these goals.

The problem with a limited menu is that it often emphasizes convenience over nutrition. Calories, and lots of them, are of course in ready supply. So if you are watching calories, there are a number of traps to avoid, if possible. Here are a few:

Trap: "I'm paying for it, so I might as well finish it."

Solutions: Leave some of it behind. Share your entree with someone else. Take part of it home in a "people bag."

Trap: "Just this once won't hurt!"

Solutions: Isn't this just like having "just one" drink? How many times have you played this game before? Once *will* hurt. Many "just this once"s can be disastrous.

Trap: "Poor me! I've done so well up to now. I *deserve* a treat."

Solutions: Find other nonfood rewards. Buy a new shirt, dress, or pair of earrings. Go to a movie. In short, reward yourself with things other than food.

To help you with your new nutritional goals, follow these guidelines when eating out:

- Avoid cream soups, quiches, gravy, and sauces.
- Avoid creamed, buttered, au gratin, breaded, and fried foods, and foods dipped in butter sauce or served with it.
- Ask for baked meat, and stay away from grilled or poached fish. And ask the waiter to "hold the butter."
- Order your salad dressings, butter, and sour cream on the side, so that you can control the amounts you use.
- Skip dessert and order fresh fruit in season.
- Ask for skim or 2 percent milk instead of whole.
- Have fruit, juice, or consommé instead of soup for a first course.

Wherever you eat out, you will obviously have a little

more control over your food in a place with a varied menu. But as a general rule you can increase the nutritive value of your meals by following our guidelines. Don't feel you're being a nuisance or causing a lot of trouble. You are paying plenty for your meals out, and you have every right to ask for what you want. If you are recovering, you need to stand right up to the waiter, waitress, or even the maître d' and ask for sauces and gravies that are prepared without alcohol. They are available, and kitchens are generally very accommodating when you make the effort and ask.

Also ask for the following:

- Whole-wheat bread, toast, or rolls instead of white.
- Salad instead of soup.
- Entrees served with green or yellow vegetables or vegetable side dishes in addition to the entree.
- Fresh fruit whenever possible.

Now with these general guidelines in mind, let's look at different types of restaurants and food-service operations and their "points of sale," so you can avoid some of the traps that can upset your program. For example, cafeterias are designed so that customers are generally encouraged to make impulse purchases.

First come the salads, which will include everything from tossed vegetables drowned in dressing, fresh or sugared fruit, jello, and other raw vegetables to perhaps plain iceberg lettuce. Next are the desserts. Here is a real trap: a wide variety of creamed, sugary foods to tempt you before you even get to the main courses.

Try to take just a tossed salad with dressing on the side, and fresh fruit. You'll get your vitamins A and C as well as fiber, and your calorie intake will be lower.

Entree choices usually include baked meat or fish as well as fried. However, even baked entrees will have been cooked in butter. Even so, they are far better choices than fried foods. Choose baked entrees without gravy, sauce, or mashed potatoes, which contain lots of butter.

The cooked vegetables usually include several green and yellow varieties. They tend to be buttered, but if you have eliminated added fat as much as possible elsewhere in the cafeteria line, then this won't matter too much. Whole-wheat bread or corn bread (both whole grains) are good. Top off your meal with a glass of milk. What you have selected is a meal that is high in food value, but relatively low in calories.

What about the fast-food places? Here are some things you should know. The places that serve fried chicken and fish have salad bars as a general rule. The problem with these places, however, is with the processed food. Buns contain large amounts of sugar because high-sugar breads do not absorb the meat juices which would give you a soggy bun. So along with a "fresh" bun you are consuming a lot of unwanted sugar.

How can you eat those french fries without catsup? Well, you probably can't. But be aware that the catsup has as much sugar as ice cream. By the way, need we remind you that those french fries are cooked in saturated fat? So are the chicken and fish.

Hamburgers are usually fried or grilled, absorbing the grease around them. You take all this information pretty much for granted. But here's an item that may surprise you and hopefully get you to think before ordering. A "shake" doesn't mean milk shake. Most shakes contain coconut oil, corn sweetener, coloring, flavoring, and minute quantities of milk, if any at all.

Those cute little fruit pies or tarts are mostly crust, with a small amount of fruit and lots of modified food starch mixed with fruit juice. So what do you do? Well, we recommend a hamburger patty, salad bar, and glass of milk. Now a lot of places obviously won't sell you the patty without the bun. Well, take it that way and then

discard the bun or eat only half of it. It's better for you.
If you can top things off with a piece of fresh fruit from
the supermarket, you're in good shape, and you will
have added to the nutrient value of the meal.

A few fast-food restaurants will offer whole-grain or
multigrain buns, which are better choices than the
usual white bun. Places serving Mexican food will have
corn tortillas, which are also whole grain. Avoid the
sour cream and use the guacamole and cheese sparingly. By doing this, you will get a fairly nutritious meal
that is low in fat, to boot. Buy an extra salad, and have
milk or juice instead of a soft drink. Again, try and stop
off for a piece of fresh fruit.

Obviously, your choices in full-service restaurants
are going to be greater. A meal that is relatively high in
nutrients would consist of a baked or broiled entree, a
baked potato with the butter and sour cream served on
the side, a vegetable, a salad (dressing on the side),
whole-grain bread, and milk.

When you eat in ethnic restaurants, you are often
faced with high-fat foods, so you need to choose carefully. As we pointed out earlier, Mexican foods that are
not fried, that contain only small amounts of cheese
and guacamole, and that are served without sour
cream are relatively low in calories. When you add a
salad and milk, you're picking up some essential
nutrients.

Italian food can be so tasty, but look out! Choose an
entree that consists primarily of pasta with a tomato-
meat sauce, a salad, and a cooked vegetable, if possible.
Added Parmesan cheese and garlic bread soaked in
butter will pile on the calories. Pizza topped with
hamburger, ham, or sausage will have more saturated
fat than pizza topped with vegetables and cheese. Try a
pizza with a thin whole-wheat crust. Add a salad (you
put on the dressing) and you're all set.

When you're in the mood for oriental food, you are in

good shape, nutritionally speaking. Stir-fried vegetables and roasted meat or poultry are relatively low in calories and high in food value. Get a salad instead of the usual egg drop soup.

The European-style restaurants—German, French, Scandinavian, etc.—are pretty high on entrees with special sauces. Not only do you have to watch the alcohol content of these sauces, but you should also be aware that they are relatively high in calories and saturated fats. Steer in the direction of baked or broiled items, along with vegetables and salads.

These same guidelines apply in other restaurants. Look for the foods that are baked or broiled without special sauces. Place the emphasis on vegetables, salads, and fresh fruits, and if you want bread, ask for whole wheat. Even if the place only has white bread, the fact that you are asking for whole wheat just might encourage them to consider stocking it in the future.

We've really been talking mostly about lunches and dinners up to now. Breakfast menus in most restaurants include poached or soft-cooked eggs, whole-wheat toast, juice, fruit, and milk. Try whole-grain pancakes or waffles; they're probably rare in most places except natural food restaurants, but they're worth the effort.

Go for whole-grain cereals such as oatmeal or Shredded Wheat. Add fruit, juice, and low-fat milk. We know this is tough on you, but avoid sweet rolls and doughnuts, which are simply loaded with grease and sugar. These items provide a very rich source of calories and nothing else.

If you thought we were giving the "roach coach" a bum rap earlier, take heart! In spite of the connotations, there are some reasonable food choices available at most of these mobile food stands. Hard-cooked eggs, salads, fresh fruit, and milk are to be found in abundance, along with the deadly sweet rolls and doughnuts. Choose wisely.

Whether you are looking for candlelight or drive-through, you should feel confident about being able to satisfy your daily protein requirement. Most places have an overabundance of it. Carbohydrates are also plentiful, but you may have a tough time getting enough whole-grain fiber, unless whole-wheat bread is available.

Restaurants that feature wide varieties of vegetables such as broccoli, carrots, peas, and green beans are also serving you vitamin A. When their salad selections include spinach and leaf lettuce as well as iceberg, then you get additional vitamin A. The lack of vitamin C and folate on many restaurant menus is of particular concern to us.

Both of these vitamins are very easily altered to the point that they are no longer active. If a restaurant holds its vegetables on steam tables for long periods of time, or if the vegetables are reheated several times, then they are no longer good sources of vitamins.

When salad greens, vegetables, and fruits are soaked in water or other solutions to preserve their crispness, they lose essential vitamins. If you are one of those persons who must eat out frequently, it would be a good idea if you stocked up on fresh fruits and vegetables elsewhere, to supplement your fast-food fare. It probably wouldn't do to haul these items into a fancy restaurant, however. Nevertheless, the point we want to make here is that you will have to be responsible for your eating, even though you may believe that the restaurant staff is there to do all the work. They are not concerned with your search for better nutrition, but they will be as helpful as possible to help you realize your goals.

Many of you have discovered that you can ask for fruit plates or special diet plates on an airplane. This is simply a matter of making the request when you book your reservation. The airline will see to it that the meal is on board. If you want to spare yourself the embarrassment of having your name blared out over the cabin intercom as the flight attendant looks for the person "who has the special meal," then make yourself known to her or him as you board. It's a little extra effort, but it's worth it.

Enjoy the candlelight. Enjoy the convenience of the "drive-through." Just reorganize your priorities so that your body benefits as much as your spirit when you eat out.

PART 3:
STICK TO
GOOD EATING
HABITS

11
Fight Stress! Eat Right!

There's no end to the amount of stress that Americans subject themselves to: changing jobs and careers, unstable relationships, unemployment and other economic pressures, and the change in lifestyles and traditional roles. These are all real "stress factories" for which there is no known cure. Traditional medical treatments are only partially effective. People frequently turn to lifestyle drugs and alcohol, as well as nicotine and caffeine, to alleviate stress.

Day in and day out, we are subjected to the pressures of producing more in less time. Perfection is expected and few allowances are made for human error. We expect our bodies to respond to pressure like machines, perhaps even better than the machines we may be operating in our daily work.

The truth is that the right amount of stress enhances your life; it sharpens your memory and learning capacity and encourages you to strive for better performance. What exactly is stress? For one thing, it's big business.

We are bombarded with advertisements promoting the use of cigarettes, alcohol, coffee, soft drinks, and high-calorie treats as rewards and relaxation. If you are "really stressed out," pain medications, antacids, sedatives, tranquilizers, and stimulants will cover up the symptoms so you can continue your present lifestyle without having to take responsibility for making the changes that might reduce or eliminate the source of stress.

When things don't go your way, the result is stress or, more accurately, distress in the body chemistry. Stress manifests itself as muscle tension and pain or is frequently experienced as worry and anxiety. The ability to change in response to stress is a primary requirement for survival. The stress reactions that are easiest to observe and to document are, of course, the physical ones. When you are "stressed," your body's chemical alarm system is sounded and messages are sent to the central nervous system. There, hormones designed to combat wear and tear on your body are activated and go to work to maintain stability as much as possible.

When stress takes the form of viruses, bacteria, or physical injury, then your body tries to decrease its sensitivity to pain and to erect a sort of "barricade." This barricade is composed of antibodies or inflamed tissue around the affected part, which helps protect the rest of your body by containing the effects of the stress.

Alcohol places a lot of stress on your body. When you drink, hormones and enzymes from your liver are secreted to detoxify the alcohol and to bring you back to normal as quickly as possible. You may have experienced one or more of these physical signs of alcohol-related stress: adrenaline "rushes," ulcers, irritable bowel, cold hands or feet, fever, and muscle tension. Perhaps you just "didn't feel well," even though this condition might not have been critical enough to create any sort of recognizable symptom.

As an alcoholic, you may have begun drinking in

response to emotional stress. By drinking you avoided dealing with stress. How many alcoholics have thought that the only way they could cope with life's problems was to drink? The truth is, of course, that it is in recovery, without alcohol, that a person begins to cope. No chemical can cover up the anxiety and make problems go away.

Your drinking and its associated stress were undoubtedly reflected in the disruption of your personal relationships. Alcohol probably raised hell with your job, your career—in short, your life. The more stress you felt, the more you relied on the alcohol to cope with it; and the more you drank, the more stress enveloped your system, creating one ugly, vicious circle. You will recall from an earlier chapter that alcohol causes the release of adrenaline, which prepares us for "fight or flight" activity and raises the blood sugar level in preparation for dealing with stress.

When you are in physical danger, your body also responds by producing adrenaline, just as if you were drinking. This adrenaline prepares your body to cope with the threat facing it. Your heart starts to beat harder and channel blood to the muscles you will need in order to flee or defend yourself.

Your appetite disappears, the blood supply to the stomach and intestines having diminished. But your blood sugar level increases so that there is energy available for whatever action is needed for your survival. If you are injured, then fluid loss is minimized in order to preserve life. Your sense of sight and sound become more acute; your thought processes are sharpened in order to increase your chances for survival.

If this stress continues for a long period of time, then just maintaining stability isn't enough, and your body may alter itself chemically and physically in order to preserve your life.

You cannot and should not avoid stress. First of all, it isn't possible to avoid stress altogether. Second, stress is one of the things that helps motivate you to make the necessary changes in your life. We call this positive kind of stress *eustress*. This eustress is the kind you feel after a good game of tennis or after running the extra mile over your set course. Eustress can be felt as the result of a passionate kiss. This kind of stress creates no conspicuous damage. But whether or not stress causes damage depends on how you react to it. When we see a coworker, friend, or family member under stress, what we really mean is that he or she is experiencing an undue amount of stress, and that he or she is responding to it in a negative or excessive way.

The stress you feel may or may not trigger noticeable physical reactions. When you are angry or frustrated, for example, you prepare your body for fighting. If you are also afraid, then you prepare to get away from the danger. In either situation, adrenaline is being released, along with other hormones, to prepare you for appropriate action.

In today's world, much stress is caused by frustration, frustration that translates into dissatisfaction with your life and a lack of respect for your own accomplishments. Many times you think, "if only something or someone would change," then life would be wonderful. When the change you hoped for doesn't take place, the combination of anger and frustration creates the desire within you to fight and make the necessary changes yourself. Fear of reprisal for being who you are, coupled with the fear of not meeting everyone else's expectations (including your own), makes you want to flee.

Many times you'll stuff your emotions, pretending that things are just "hunky-dory," or at least tolerable, when in fact your insides are churning like a volcano about to explode. Many people become so adept at *not* feeling that they really don't experience appropriate emotions. This only serves to strengthen the denial of a particular problem or situation. Modern-day stressors are frequently nonphysical, chronic, and unrelieved. Your body stays in a constant state of crisis.

Your body was designed to handle stress immediately and to use the hormones released, *not* to stay in the crisis mode for any length of time. When your mind and spirit fail to handle stress, then your body is called on to take the heat, and the physical symptoms of stress appear.

The types of symptoms will vary from one person to the next and will have a lot to do with which body organ or system is most vulnerable. We're going to list just some of the most common physical symptoms related to stress. You can add to the list from your own experiences:

General irritability
Depression
Increased heart rate and blood pressure
Dryness of the throat and mouth
Impulsive behavior and/or emotional
    instability
Poor concentration and general disorientation
Weakness or dizziness
Overpowering urge to cry, run, hide, or
    disappear
Chronic fatigue
Insomnia and/or nightmares
Anxiety not focused on any one thing
Fear without specific reason
Overreaction to small sounds or sudden light
Emotional tension or feeling "keyed up"
High-pitched speech or laughter
Grinding or clenching teeth
Inability to relax or enjoy play
Excessive perspiration, frequent urination
Diarrhea, indigestion, stomach queasiness
Migraine headaches

Premenstrual syndrome, irregular menstrual
  periods
Pain in the neck or lower back (muscle
  tension)
Increased smoking
Increased coffee or sugar consumption
Increased use of prescription or over-the-
  counter medications
Frequent colds, flu, and other infections
Frequent absenteeism due to real illness or
  just "not feeling well"
Increased allergy symptoms, or the
  appearance of allergies where there were
  none before
Changes in food-consumption patterns

That's a lot to attribute to stress! By "changes in food-consumption patterns," we really mean the tendency to avoid food when you are under stress, especially if there is a physical injury or illness.

If you are experiencing extreme emotional trauma, you are also probably not very hungry. Your body has enough reserves to carry you through for several days without food, so you shouldn't force yourself to eat. But if your lack of appetite continues, then a one-a-day supplement might be in order to help your body maintain its immune system.

But some of you may be saying at this point, "Not me! When I'm under stress, I eat like a horse!" Well, part of that syndrome originates in childhood. You know, when you were little, you calmed down when you were handed a cookie, some ice cream, or other treats. Of course, what was really happening was that your parent or sitter was feeding the hurt, angry, or otherwise stressed-out kid, instead of giving him love.

But the adult habit forms when you provide yourself with "comfort" foods. Eating these foods gives a sense of relief because blood is temporarily shunted away from the brain and nerves and toward the digestive system, altering your reaction to the stress.

When you eat to reduce stress, you feel more relaxed, your appetite increases, and you eat even more. Well, you can see what this can lead to. Excessive weight gain is not only possible but probable with this kind of eating. It is better to engage in an activity or exercise to relieve stress than to eat.

If your diet is high in fat, sugar, and especially cholesterol, it adds to your physical and emotional stress. When you select "empty calorie" foods or eat poorly prepared foods, you also increase your level of stress. Interestingly enough, people who overeat when they are under stress tend to select foods that are devoid of nutrients and high in fat and sugar. We see a pretty clear connection between a person's decreased ability to handle stress and a poor diet. The best prevention is to eat regularly and include a wide variety of nutrient-dense foods.

Here are some guidelines for making nutritional changes that will help you cope with stress. As with all guidelines, it might be a good idea for you to post them in places like your kitchen or eating area.

- Establish regular mealtimes and adhere to them.
- Set aside a minimum of 30 minutes for each meal, and use the entire period of time.
- Eliminate eating while driving, watching TV, or reading.
- Eat consciously. Be aware of what you are eating.
- Chew your food slowly and savor its taste.
- Eat foods that provide needed nutrients.
- Eliminate "empty calorie" foods.
- Reduce caffeine intake.
- Allow for small amounts of treats or favorite foods once or twice a week.
- Don't binge!

Keep these guidelines firmly in mind as you combat stress. Recent medical and nutritional research has proven that stressful situations such as surgery, burns, or severe accidents can be alleviated with larger amounts of specific vitamins and minerals. Vitamins A, B_1, B_2, and C, niacin, zinc, potassium, and possibly copper, sulphur, and phosphorus are all needed in larger amounts than usual when physical stress is present.

If a person's immune system is affected by infection or chronic disease, then larger amounts of vitamins A, C, B_{12}, B_6, niacin, folate, iron, zinc, and protein are needed. A visit to any drugstore today will show what impact stress in general is having on the buying public. There is a wide selection of products designed to help people cope with stress. As enticing as the idea may be that you can just pop a few of these concoctions to ease life's anxieties, there is no scientific evidence to support the use of these supplements for emotional stress.

As a matter of fact, recent research shows that the nutritional needs of a person under emotional stress can be met, in most situations, with a one-a-day supplement. These findings directly contradict popular theories about vitamin "megadoses," which may actually increase stress by creating nutritional imbalances.

Recovering alcoholics must learn that it is in their nature to crave excitement. You are prone to try to "live on the edge" all the time. You will attempt to do as much as you can in a short period of time. You tend to do too many things at once, rarely stopping to "smell the roses" along the way. You want to make up for all the time that was lost while you were drinking, and before you know it, you may become what we call an "adrenaline junkie."

These "adrenaline junkies" work in high-pressure jobs, rolling from one crisis to the next, avoiding dull, repetitive tasks. The recovering person who is also an "adrenaline junkie" loves romantic adventures, late-night meetings, skydiving, hang gliding, risky deals of all kinds, as well as changing jobs and romantic partners frequently—anything and everything to keep the level of excitement high.

Adrenaline, you recall, produces a sense of well-being, of being high or euphoric, efficient, sharp, and alert. Learning to live without kicking in the adrenaline is as great a challenge for the addictive person as is learning to live his life without alcohol. The difference, of course, is that you produce adrenaline yourself.

In some instances, your very survival may depend on adrenaline, so you don't want to eliminate it entirely. However, slowing down and enjoying life at a more even pace establishes a different lifestyle, which will fit right in with your overall goals of recovery.

Some specific changes can be made to help you control your stress levels and thus reduce the temptation to run on adrenaline and become an "adrenaline junkie." Be aware of your maximum stress level and of the body signals that indicate change is needed or that stress is building. Learn to balance mental exertion with physical activity, such as our old standby, aerobic exercise. If your stress relates to physical activity, then for goodness' sake change the activity. If you have strained a muscle in your running program, change to bicycling or swimming, for example.

Learn to relax completely and to forget your work and its related stress. Oh, we know that's easier said than done, but you must try. Getting involved in physical exercise is a dynamite way to put the day's cares behind you.

Don't put more energy into a project than is necessary for producing the desired results. Setting reasonable goals for each day's work will help you gain a sense of achievement. You won't feel stressed because you didn't get everything done at once. We could not end this chapter on stress without encouraging you again to take time for meals and relaxation at regular intervals throughout the day.

Set limits for yourself, and combine them with proper nutrition. This will be a great step forward in your program of recovery. Remind yourself that you are already an addictive person who tends to do too much too soon, that you are a prime candidate for becoming an "adrenaline junkie." Stress management is possible for you. Your battle cry is "Fight stress! Eat right!"

12
Exercise and Nutrition: A Formula for Recovery

Exercise, along with good nutrition, is important for good health. In this chapter, let's look at how eating right and exercising work together for the recovering person.

For those of you concerned about your weight, aerobic exercise increases the rate at which the body burns calories, not just while you're exercising, but all the time. In the beginning, you may find that 5 minutes of daily exercise is all you can tolerate. And why not? If you don't use a muscle or an organ, it gets weaker and less functional.

But your goal is to work up to 20 minutes a day, even though we realize that may be pushing you to the limits of your endurance. In order to lose weight and maintain your desired weight, you must exercise regularly for 20 minutes at a time, six days a week.

We, your authors, favor aerobic exercise and jogging. Both of these increase your heart rate and oxygen use. Also good are swimming (laps), bicycling, jumping rope, and fast walking.

Aerobic exercise maintains or improves muscle tone and decreases the accumulation of body fat. You will remember that body fat increases with age. Without exercise, therefore, your percentage of body fat can double or even triple, even though your weight might not change that much.

Worse, muscles that are not used shrink and are replaced with fatty tissue. When you exercise, you improve your blood circulation, lower your blood pressure, and decrease the amount of fat in the blood, which means lower levels of cholesterol and triglycerides. Exercise strengthens your heart so it can pump more blood with each beat and improves the oxygen-carrying capacity of your blood. Not bad for just a few minutes a day?

Let's look at what fuel your body needs to function. Fuel for muscles is obtained from the carbohydrates, fats, and proteins you consume. The most efficient fuel (and, incidentally, the one that supplies 50 to 60 percent of your calories) is carbohydrates.

FUEL FOR EXERCISE
Carbohydrates

Carbohydrates include simple sugars, such as those found in fruits and sweets, and complex carbohydrates, chains formed of simple sugars, such as the starches in vegetables and grains. Simple carbohydrates provide quick energy but are used up quickly because they are easily digested and converted into glucose.

Complex carbohydrates take 4 to 6 hours to be processed by the body and converted into glucose. While this is happening, you get a steady stream of blood sugar into your system. The carbohydrates that are not needed for energy still have a purpose; they get stored as body starch, providing a ready reserve when you need a boost.

Most of this body starch (about two-thirds) is stored

in your muscles, and the remainder, in your liver. A marathon runner accumulates enough of these reserves to last through the hours of grueling activity that constitute a race.

Not all folks are marathoners, however. Fortunately, your body adapts to your level of activity, so that your muscles get enough oxygen, no matter what you are doing. Remember, we call this stored body starch glycogen, and the reason it is stored in the liver is to sustain you when you go for long periods of time without food, such as at night.

A lot of runners will do a "glycogen load-up" before a race in order to deplete the stores of this body starch. First, they will maintain a low-carbohydrate diet for several days before the event to force their bodies to use up their ready reserves. A day or two prior to the event, the runner will go on a "carbo-binge," eating huge amounts of grain products, starchy vegetables, spaghetti, and other pastas. The purpose of this is to force the body to overload on glycogen, thus providing bountiful stores of energy when the race takes place. Other sports use this training technique, too. What's important to remember is that this formula works because the athlete is training on a daily basis.

However, most people who exercise more casually, then get fired up, and decide to run a long race—say, a 10K—won't benefit much from this carbo-loading process. The exercise has to be more consistent.

Fat

Fat is stored in your muscles, under the skin, and around internal organs. The trained athlete's body has adapted in such a way that it can use fat for energy during exercise. If an athlete is participating in endurance work, up to 75 percent of his or her energy can come from fat instead of carbohydrates. During a marathon, for example, studies have shown that muscle-fat stores in the marathoner's body can decrease by 30 percent or more.

However, for average runners, fat is *not* used as a source of energy, even when they exercise a little more than usual. The point of exercising for you (and frankly for most of us) is to improve muscle tone and decrease the overall percentage of fat in the body.

Protein

Although proteins are the building blocks for muscle, there isn't much evidence to support the use of protein as an energy source for exercising. You get extra muscle strength from using the protein, rather than from consuming it in larger quantities. If you're a weight lifter, for example, the maximum amount of muscle mass that you can add in one week is 1 pound. So, if you simply add 2 extra ounces of protein in the form of meat, poultry, or fish each day, you will get the protein you need for your weight training.

If you exercise 20 minutes a day, you won't need extra protein to build muscle. The amount of protein in the average American diet (which overemphasizes protein anyway) is more than enough to supply your needs. In other words, two 8-ounce glasses of milk and 4 to 6 ounces of meat, fish, or poultry per day will supply the average person with adequate protein.

Amino acids are the building blocks of protein. Some people take amino acid supplements in purified form to reduce the amount of work the body must do to digest protein. Well, as logical as it may sound, the facts don't support this practice very well. Why? Because as proteins are digested, amino acids are released into your body and absorbed from the small intestine. From there, they are transported to the body tissues that need them.

As you will recall from an earlier chapter where we introduced "receptor sites," these amino acids attach to specific sites in the intestinal lining—sites designed for each amino acid.

When you supply your body with purified amino acids, these receptor sites fill up very quickly. When there is no more room at the site, the unabsorbed amino acids are eliminated from your body.

Ideally, you will get all the nutrients you need from eating nutrient-dense foods instead of junk foods. Taking a vitamin pill might lull you into thinking that all your nutritional needs are being met, so your calories can come from anywhere. Many studies have been done on the nutritional needs of Olympic athletes, with an eye toward improving performance through vitamin and mineral supplementation. The idea behind all this is to supply extra amounts of the vitamins that affect energy production and therefore endurance. However, there is no conclusive evidence that vitamin supplements improve endurance.

Minerals

The relationship of minerals to exercise should be understood not only by the recovering person, but by the general public as well. Calcium occupies center stage because of the attention being paid to osteoporosis. Lack of exercise is almost guaranteed to result in a loss of calcium from the bone. So, the amount of calcium that is absorbed in the bones could depend on your exercise habits. With adequate calcium, bones reach their maximum density at approximately age 35.

If you have abused alcohol, nicotine, and caffeine, you have specifically been interfering with your body's calcium absorption and the depositing of calcium in your bones. The recovering person, therefore, is likely to be embarking on his or her exercise program with a calcium deficit. Dairy foods (with the exception of ice cream) are the most concentrated sources of calcium in our systems.

You all recognize that iron is essential in helping your blood carry oxygen. Women who are menstruating, whether they exercise or not, need to make sure they are getting enough iron, either from food or from supplements. Stay away from megadoses, however, because they can be toxic. Men generally get the iron they need from their food.

You have undoubtedly heard a great deal about electrolyte supplements, sodium and potassium. Food and water will provide all the electrolytes you need for regular exercise, and even for a special event such as a marathon. *Stay away from salt tablets: they can be dangerous.*

Water

Now, here's the surprise in this recovery-and-exercise formula. The critical element for those of you who are athletes, as well as for those of you who are determined to take up and stick with aerobics, is water.

No surprise, you say? OK, but let's review just how important water is to your body. First of all, it's the main component of your body, 60 percent of the whole including cells, urine, sweat, blood, lymph, hormones, and enzymes. It performs vital functions for you. It transports nutrients, provides the medium for chemical reactions, and, like the radiator in your car, regulates body temperature. This last function is pretty important when you're exercising, because your muscles heat up during sustained exercise. Evaporation of sweat is your body's primary way of releasing heat. If you are dehydrated, your endurance can be greatly affected. Of course, whether you exercise or not, you need a certain amount of water daily. The more you exercise, the more fluid you need to replace what you are losing through exercise.

Fluids can be obtained from both food and water, but you pick up a lot of calories from the fluids in foods, unless you are drinking liquids such as milk, juice, or soup. If you're concerned about your weight, then getting water from food instead of drinking it also means eating lots of calories that you certainly don't need.

The recommended water intake for the average person is 1½ quarts a day. This doesn't include any coffee, tea, soda, or other caffeinated beverages. Why? Because these drinks act as diuretics and increase the amount of water lost through urination. By the way, when you drink more water, you tend to drink less coffee, tea, and soda.

Now let's wrap up some points about your exercise-and-recovery plan. You've heard the expression, "hitting the wall"? This is a reaction that occurs when muscles start to run on glycogen only. You see, the glycogen that is in a muscle before you start to exercise stays in that muscle until it is used up. It can't migrate from one muscle to another, even though another muscle might need it desperately. So when those fat and extra glycogen stores are used up, and the muscle is down to running on its glycogen only, the glycogen stores are quickly depleted. Once these ready reserves are gone, you start "hitting the wall" with sore, painful, uncoordinated muscles.

You can push yourself at this point and continue to exercise, but the muscle tissue itself starts to be used for energy, and every movement becomes extremely painful. By the way, if you exercise in hot weather, you will use up more glycogen than if you exercise in mild or cold weather.

Blood sugar is a primary source of fuel for your muscles. You maintain your blood sugar levels by converting liver glycogen into blood sugar (glucose). If, during exercise, you deplete your liver glycogen, you will feel all the reactions of hypoglycemia (low blood sugar). You begin to feel faint, dizzy, shaky, confused, uncoordinated, and clammy. Your brain just can't function properly, so you must eat something to replace the lost glucose for your brain. If you eat immediately, the recovery takes about 20 to 30 minutes.

This reaction is referred to by athletes as "bonking," and they will take nourishment during competition to lessen the chances of a "bonk." It's possible to "hit the wall" and "bonk" at the same time, but the big difference is that recovering from "hitting the wall" usually takes 24 hours, with muscle soreness that can stay with you for several days or more.

Oxygen is required for your body to burn glycogen and fat efficiently, just like the furnace in your home. The peak rate at which your body can take in and use oxygen is determined by your genetic makeup and varies from one person to the next. With training, you can increase this rate. Endurance increases with the length of time you can exercise at pretty close to capacity.

Exercising with sufficient oxygen is called aerobic exercise. Your most efficient use of oxygen occurs when your pulse rate doesn't go over 130 beats per minute. When you start to breathe hard and pant, lactic acid begins to build up; your body is trying to get more air. An important process is happening here. When glycogen is converted to glucose and then used for energy, a substance called pyruvate is formed.

When there is plenty of oxygen available to your body, pyruvate is converted to carbon dioxide and water and is easily eliminated through your lungs. However, if you suffer an "oxygen deficiency" in the muscles, this same pyruvate is converted to lactic acid, which accumulates in the muscles and then moves into the bloodstream.

What's so bad about that? Plenty! The lactic acid interferes with muscle contraction and relaxation. This makes it extremely difficult for muscles to move, and the result is a real feeling of fatigue. When lactic acid levels build to a higher concentration, then your muscles may stop functioning altogether. You begin to lose control over your muscles. They become increasingly painful and may even cramp. When there is oxygen available, this lactic acid we've been talking about is converted into pyruvate and then into carbon dioxide and water.

The use of steroids has made the news in the past months, since it is the "in" thing among body builders. A steroid user's goal is to get a beautiful body now and not worry about the consequences. But steroids merely make your body retain water, giving the illusion of larger muscles. In normal doses, the effects of steroids are no different than those achieved by regular workouts.

The side effects are bone loss, decreased functioning of the adrenal and pituitary glands, and decreased functioning of the testicles. Not such good news, after all. That's a high price to pay for the short-term pleasure of appearing to have more muscle.

So, recovery and nutrition, exercise and feeling good about yourself again are all part of your life of sobriety. As you progress toward wellness, your diet and nutrition will become second nature to you.

Men and women, dust off those Nikes! You can find an exercise program that's just right for you. As Snuffy Smith of the comics says, "Time's a-wastin'!"

13
The Recovery Connection

Well, this is it! We've sorted, sifted, counted, baked, broiled, and rechanneled our thinking for the last 12 chapters. We're near the end, or is it the beginning? For what we have tried to introduce into your life of recovery is the importance of examining the way in which you may have neglected one of the fundamental aspects of a joyous, sober life. Food! How it looks, how it's prepared, how it tastes, and how it can provide you with the foundation of a healthier and happier life.

Recovery is a holistic process, in which no element necessarily has priority over another. All of your energies seem to be channeled into the physical, mental, spiritual, and social areas of your life that alcohol has disrupted or nearly destroyed. What we want to do is to add another dimension: the way you think and feel and act around the foods you prepare and eat.

Face it. When alcohol was the prime mover in your life, food and its nutrient values, preparation, and consumption took a back seat. What interested you most was booze. Well, that's behind you now and hopefully will stay that way.

Your top priority is maintaining sobriety. Without it you have nothing! Attitude is the most crucial factor in your health, and exercise is second. What you eat is, of course, affected by your attitude. You might very well feel guilty because you find yourself relying on convenience foods rather than cooking everything from scratch. If you're a perfectionist, then all of this nutrition business may look like the key you've been seeking to some "magic cure" in your recovery.

Well, it isn't! It *is* a vital link that you need to examine carefully before deciding to risk making changes in the way you have felt about food and your physical condition. When we emphasize exercise in this book, we are not trying to get you out running five or six miles a day, but rather to get you into an aerobic exercise pattern of 20 minutes every day. This would be a great goal for you to set yourself and *reach!*

You don't have to be compulsive about any of this, but rather set yourself a realistic goal and then work up to the ideal. Two to five minutes a day, but *every* day, is a great way for you to start. Don't worry about what someone else is doing. Just take care of yourself and relish the small accomplishments that you attain. You'll get there two and three minutes at a time. Trust us!

Plan your exercise around other activities instead of at a specific time each day. Be practical. After all, if you are working overtime, then a rigid 6:00 P.M. workout time isn't going to hold up, is it? What's important is that you find the two to five minutes either before work or after. The sense of accomplishment will spur you on to begin increasing your time and placing more importance on exercise.

The next highest priority for you is to always keep in mind the nutrient values of the foods you eat. Too often, particularly in your active drinking stage, calories were what got your attention. Well, look at what we have been discussing in these pages. If fruits and raw vegetables have not been prominent in your diet, then for goodness' sake make them!

Start by adding the vegetables that appear most often in social situations or when eating out. You know, at your next party or gathering, pass up the chips and dips, and head for the veggie trays. When you are in a place that offers a salad bar, use it.

You can try small amounts of two or three vegetables and then add some of the things that you swore you would "never touch with a 10-foot pole." Surprise yourself! Alcohol has impaired everything from your sense of taste and smell right down to your liver and stomach, so you may not even realize what many vegetables taste like.

If fruits are difficult for you, then start with just one that you like and use it as a dessert. And if you really need help, mix it with a little yogurt or perhaps some vanilla ice cream. The point is, try it.

If fruits and vegetables are not a problem, all the better. We know, it's whole-grain breads and cereals you really can't stand. Well, go back to the chapter on dietary change and implement some of the steps we suggested for getting used to the texture and flavor of whole grains. Work on brown rice, for example.

Remember that for most of your life you have probably been using white bread, white rice, and mashed potatoes. Expect a little discomfort from intestinal gas when you start increasing the amount of fiber in your diet. As you slowly add fiber to your diet, this discomfort will pass. You will find yourself wondering why you didn't eat like this a long time ago.

Your recovery will depend on your continuing to play "Sherlock Holmes" with foods. Look at labels, be very aware of sugar and fat content, etc. The trick is to choose foods that are as high in nutrient value as possible, without loading up on unwanted calories.

You can do it. And don't start pouting, either! Eating

something that really turns you off just because it's good for you, doesn't do a whole lot for your positive attitude. Quite the contrary, it's likely to make you feel downright defiant about all this "new diet stuff." We don't want that, do we?

Keep in mind (post it up on a kitchen wall) that you are trying to reduce the amount of high-fat and sugary foods you eat and to increase the amount of complex carbohydrates in your diet. If you load up on protein, you will also get the fat that always accompanies meat, fish, and poultry. Complex carbohydrates don't have this disadvantage.

Assume responsibility for the way you eat and for what you eat. This is as much a part of your overall recovery program as the other elements that relate directly to your sobriety. There is no perfect plan that we know of, no specific diet that will lead you into the promised land. What we do know is that you can use the tools we have provided to make drastic and necessary changes in your diet.

The so-called facts about diets and food that apply to, say, 60 percent of the general population who are normal and healthy will not necessarily apply to the person in recovery from substance abuse. The idea is to try out the suggestions we have given you. Some you will like, others you will dislike, but all are worth your attention. Find what works best for you. It's that simple.

Seek guidance from knowledgeable health-care professionals on any physical problems that need to be addressed, before you tackle any abrupt dietary changes. We have assumed that you have entered recovery with fairly poor eating habits. There are those of you, of course, who have entered into sobriety with good or even excellent nutritional habits, and we applaud you.

The physical recovery of individuals with good eating habits is likely to be several steps ahead of that of individuals who rarely ate at all or became "fast-food freaks." For those of you with good nutritional habits, try to find points in the foregoing chapters that will help you fine-tune your diet for recovery.

If you are new to good nutrition, then take it just like your sobriety: one step at a time! Don't try to do it all at once. It is our hope that you will take pride in getting in touch with your body and its needs, physical and emotional alike.

Finally, feeling good about what you are doing is as important as actually doing it. The following chapter offers you a basic set of recipes to start working with. Experiment, learn, and savor the idea of good food, good health, and good recovery!

14
Recipes for a Healthful Recovery

STORING FOODS

Fresh Fruits and Vegetables

- Purchase only the amount of fresh fruits and vegetables you can use in a short period of time.
- Most fresh vegetables should be stored in the crisper in plastic bags or in a cool place (40°F). (Potatoes should be stored in a cool, dark place, but not in the refrigerator. A brown paper bag placed away from heat sources is fine.)
- Before storing vegetables in the refrigerator, remove tops from carrots and beets, wash off dirt, and remove decayed or bruised areas. Drain well before storing.
- Ripe fruit should not be mixed with vegetables in the crisper. The fruit gives off ethylene gas, which causes toughening of some vegetables and a bitter taste in others. Cabbage-family vegetables (cabbage, broccoli, brussels sprouts, cauliflower, kale, and kohlrabi) will pass their strong odors on to

other vegetables, so keep them in separate plastic bags.

- Tomatoes and other fruits are best stored at room temperature until ripe and then placed in the refrigerator.
- Onions and garlic should be stored in containers where air can circulate (baskets, mesh bags, or perforated boxes) at room temperature.

Grains

- Whole-grain breads are best refrigerated. If they are not going to be used within a short period of time, freeze the extra. Bread keeps well in the refrigerator for approximately a week and a half.
- Cereals keep well at room temperature in closed containers. If cereal grains for cooking have been purchased in bulk, place them in closed metal or plastic containers, and store away from heat sources. Some vitamins are lost when grains are exposed to light, so glass containers on open shelves are not a good idea. If you are not going to use cereals within a month of purchase, storing them in closed containers in the refrigerator is probably a good idea.

Dairy Products

- Milk needs to be placed is the coldest part of the refrigerator. In most refrigerators, the bottom is the coldest since cold air is heavier than warm. The door shelves are slightly warmer than other parts of the refrigerator and are therefore the best place to keep cheese.

Meat, Fish, Poultry, and Eggs

- Some refrigerators have a specified place for storing meat, fish, and poultry. In general, these items need to be kept in the coldest part of the refrigerator. Fish should be frozen if it will not be used within two days of purchase, and meat and poultry should be cooked within four days of purchase or frozen until needed. Cooked meats, fish, and poultry freeze well and can be thawed for quick meals.

Herbs and Spices

- Herbs and spices become rancid if they are kept near heat sources. Place them away from the range, heat register, and sunlight.
- If you use these seasonings infrequently or in very small amounts, try purchasing them at stores that sell herbs in bulk and will sell you an ounce or less. The flavor of fresh herbs makes the extra effort of getting them this way worthwhile.

REVISING RECIPES FOR HEALTH

In most recipes, the amount of sugar content can be reduced by a third to a half without significantly changing the flavor. If the family is accustomed to the full amount of sugar in a recipe, reducing it gradually might be a good idea.

Salt levels can easily be reduced in foods that contain herbs and spices. In foods where salt is the primary flavor, reduce it gradually until you and others become accustomed to the flavor of the food itself. People who have used less salt for long periods of time find foods that are "normally" salted to be too salty. They also learn to taste the salt that occurs naturally in meat, fish, poultry, eggs, and some vegetables. The flavors of many foods are very subtle; until you eliminate or reduce the amount of added salt, you cannot experience them.

But even those who do not care for a lot of salt find that certain foods are hard to eat without it. The foods that are hardest to accept without salt are bread and cooked cereal. Adding cinnamon to cereal might take the place of salt, but most people don't want bread with added herbs or spices on a regular basis. Reducing the salt elsewhere and using regular bread with salt added is fine for most people, even if they have doctor's orders to restrict salt and sodium.

Reducing the fat content of recipes or using oil instead of shortening, margarine, or butter significantly alters the texture of some foods. Making the changes gradually might be necessary. Substituting low-fat cheeses and milk for full-fat cheese and whole milk is a fairly easy adjustment to make. Skim milk in coffee instead of coffee creamer (which is made of coconut oil and corn syrup) might seem like a real hassle at first. Later you take the taste for granted. For those who like the fat on meat and poultry or who really notice the difference in flavor, trimming off all the visible fat is a major change. Using herbs and spices helps smooth the transition and keeps you from feeling so deprived.

Vegetable oil makes biscuits and pie crusts very different from what you are used to. For that reason, you might choose to use shortening in those two items and have them less often. The texture of other foods when oil is used instead of shortening might be softer and less crisp. Most people can accept soft cookies or muffins as well as crusty ones and find that in the long run having them made with oil makes little difference to them.

Increasing fiber in the diet can be done in many ways. Leave the skin on apples, pears, cucumber, and tomatoes. Use oatmeal or oat bran as the extender in meat, salmon, or turkey loaf instead of cracker crumbs. Make burritos and tostados with beans instead of meat. Top yogurt with bran, sunflower seeds, or chopped fresh apples or pears. Use whole fruit instead of juice; not only will there be more fiber, but it will be more filling and less will be consumed. Use popcorn as a snack. Eat baked potato skins. Add cooked or grated raw carrots, cabbage, celery, and zucchini to meat loaf. Use cooked legumes as part of the protein in soups, casseroles, and fish or poultry salads.

The following recipes cover a wide variety of possibilities, with everything from the very simple to the gourmet touched upon. The special sauces and soups may be more complicated than you want to tackle. Look for the recipes that fit your lifestyle, budget, and schedule.

When we make changes in our diets, especially when we eliminate sauces and rich foods, we tend to think that we are being deprived of something very special. We even get to thinking that we are being mistreated. The truth is that each food has a flavor and texture that is unique and interesting. When we cover up these flavors and textures with special sauces and seasonings, we mask the innate qualities of that food. Try preparing some foods, especially fruits and vegetables, plain, and learn to appreciate their unique flavors.

HOMEMADE SEASONINGS

All-Purpose Herb Mix

2 teaspoons onion powder
¼ teaspoon black pepper
½ teaspoon garlic powder
1 teaspoon dry mustard
1 teaspoon paprika
½ teaspoon thyme
2 teaspoons basil
½ teaspoon parsley flakes
½ teaspoon marjoram
¾ teaspoon salt

Mix all ingredients together and store in a jar in the refrigerator.

Hot Chili Powder

1 large dried red chili (can be purchased
   in Spanish food section)
2 teaspoons paprika
2 teaspoons black pepper
1 tablespoon leaf oregano
1 tablespoon leaf basil
2 teaspoons cumin seeds
1 teaspoon coriander
½ teaspoon garlic powder

Mix all ingredients together in blender or food processor until finely ground. Store in an airtight container. *Note:* This mixture is much hotter than the chili powder sold in spice sections. Use it sparingly. Cumin is the herb that has the most bite to it. If a milder chili powder is desired, reduce the amount of cumin.

Saltless "Salt"

2 teaspoons thyme
2 teaspoons savory
2 teaspoons sage
2 teaspoons basil
1 tablespoon marjoram
¼ teaspoon garlic

Mix all ingredients together in blender or food processor. Store in an airtight container.

Poultry Seasoning

2 tablespoons marjoram
2 tablespoons parsley flakes
2 tablespoons savory
1 tablespoon sage
1½ teaspoons thyme
¼ teaspoon nutmeg
¼ teaspoon black pepper

Mix all ingredients together in blender or food processor. Store in an airtight container.

QUICK MEALS

Bean Burrito

⅓ cup pinto beans, drained
1 tablespoon Homemade Salsa (recipe
    follows)
1 whole-wheat tortilla
Chopped onion (optional)
Garlic powder (optional)

Place beans and salsa down center of tortilla. Sprinkle with onion and garlic powder if desired. Fold both edges over center and warm in a 350°F oven or a microwave.

Serves 1

Homemade Salsa

3 fresh chilies or jalapeño peppers,
    roasted and peeled, *or* 1 small can
    green chili
3 tomatillos *or* 1 medium green tomato,
    chopped
1 bunch green onions, chopped
2 medium tomatoes, chopped
1 medium avocado, chopped
15 sprigs cilantro *or* parsley
½ cup lime juice
2 tablespoons olive oil
1 teaspoon garlic powder
1 teaspoon ground cumin
½ teaspoon salt

Mix all ingredients together in blender or food processor, until coarsely chopped. Chill before serving.

Makes 1½ cups

Chips and Dip

½ can pinto beans, drained
½ teaspoon cumin powder
1 tablespoon canned green chili
2 tablespoons tomato sauce
Corn chips or corn tortillas

Place first four ingredients in blender or food processor and mix thoroughly. Heat over low heat, stirring to keep from sticking and burning. Serve with corn chips or corn tortillas that have been toasted in the oven. The combination of beans and corn makes a complete protein.

Serves 2

Fruited Yogurt

8 ounces plain low-fat yogurt
1 tablespoon frozen fruit juice concentrate
½ cup unsweetened frozen or fresh fruit

Mix all ingredients in blender for a quick breakfast or snack.

Serves 1

Mini Pizza

1 whole-wheat tortilla
1 fresh tomato, sliced *or* 3–4 tablespoons
    tomato sauce
¼ cup grated cheese
Garlic powder
Onion powder
Italian seasoning

Place fresh tomato slices or tomato sauce on tortilla. Top with grated cheese and sprinkle with garlic powder, onion powder, and Italian seasoning. Place under broiler until the cheese is melted.

Serves 1

Pita Pockets

3½ ounces water-packed tuna or chicken
1 rib celery, chopped
1 small grated carrot
1 small tomato, chopped
2 teaspoons low-fat plain yogurt or
    mayonnaise
1 pita bread

Combine tuna or chicken, vegetables, and yogurt or mayonnaise. Cut pita bread in half to form pockets and stuff with filling. Alfalfa sprouts or lettuce may also be added.

Serves 1

SOUPS

Beef and Bean Soup

1 pound soup or neck bones
1½ quarts water
3 medium potatoes, diced
3 medium carrots, diced
1 medium onion, diced
2 ribs celery, chopped
2 cups canned pinto beans
1 medium can tomatoes *or* 3 fresh
    tomatoes
Salt, pepper, and oregano to taste

Cook the soup or neck bones in an electric slow cooker with 1½ quarts water until meat pulls away from the bone (about 3 hours at low temperature). Remove the bones. Add potatoes, carrots, onion, and celery, and cook until tender (about 1 hour at medium high temperature). Add beans, tomatoes, and seasoning.

Serves 6–8

Vegetarian Chili

1 cup each pinto, navy, and kidney beans
1 medium onion
2 cloves garlic
2 teaspoons chili powder
1 teaspoon salt
½ teaspoon black pepper
2 16-ounce cans tomatoes *or* 8 medium
    fresh tomatoes
2 cups cooked rice or barley
2 tablespoons vegetable oil
Whole-wheat bread or crackers

Soak the beans overnight, pour off the soaking water, and add fresh water to cover. Cook in electric slow cooker with onion, garlic, and seasonings for 6 hours. Add the tomatoes, rice or barley, and oil. Serve with whole-wheat bread or crackers.

Note: Adding baking soda to dried beans decreases their gas-forming properties, but it also destroys a number of vitamins. Soaking the beans, pouring off the soaking water, and adding fresh water has the same effect with less loss of nutrients.

Serves 8–10

"Must Go" Soup

3–4 medium potatoes, diced
1 medium onion, diced
1 cup lentils
Leftover vegetables
Salt and pepper to taste
1 tablespoon vegetable oil (optional)
Pinch of ground cloves (optional)
Whole-wheat crackers *or* toasted corn
    tortillas

Cook potatoes, onion, and lentils in 1 quart water over medium heat until tender, about 30 minutes. Add leftover vegetables and seasonings. A small amount of vegetable oil and a pinch of ground cloves will make the soup taste richer. Serve with whole-wheat crackers or toasted corn tortillas to provide a complete protein.

Serves 6–8

Creamy Potato Soup

5 medium potatoes, diced
1 medium onion
1 clove garlic
⅓ cup powdered milk
3 cups milk
½ teaspoon salt
¼ teaspoon pepper
2 teaspoons butter or margarine

Cook potatoes, onion, and garlic in enough water to cover, until tender. If there is a lot of water in the pot, add powdered milk, stirring it in gradually to convert the cooking water into milk. Add fluid milk, seasonings, and butter or margarine.

Note: Leftover vegetables such as carrots, peas, broccoli, and spinach can be added for variation. For those on a tight budget, cooking broccoli stalks, blending them, and adding them to this recipe makes a good cream of broccoli soup.

Serves 6–8

Spinach Soup

1 pound russet potatoes, diced
1 cup sliced carrots
1 large onion, diced
1 cup water
½ teaspoon salt
2 cups chicken broth
1 bunch fresh spinach *or* 1 10-ounce
    package frozen spinach
1 cup milk
1 tablespoon butter
Pepper to taste

Combine potatoes, carrots, onion, water, salt, and broth.
Bring to a boil, reduce heat, cover, and simmer until
vegetables are tender. Rinse spinach well and break off
stems, if fresh is being used. Add spinach to pot, cover,
and cook until spinach is wilted. Puree in blender until
smooth, stir in milk, and heat. Spoon into bowls, add a
small amount of butter to each bowl, and sprinkle with
pepper.

Serves 8

Tomato Soup with Tarragon

1 tablespoon oil
1 large onion, diced
4 large tomatoes, quartered
4 cups chicken broth
1 tablespoon crumbled tarragon leaves
1 teaspoon thyme leaves
½ bay leaf
Salt to taste

Heat oil in heavy skillet and cook onion in it until transparent. Stir in tomatoes, chicken broth, herbs, and salt. Bring to boil, then reduce heat and simmer until thickened, about 25 minutes. Remove bay leaf and puree in blender until smooth. Warm and serve immediately or chill and serve cold.

Serves 6–8

Creamy Tomato and Carrot Soup

1 medium onion, chopped
¼ cup oil
¾ pound carrots, chopped
1 medium tart apple
2 teaspoons minced garlic *or* ¼ teaspoon
    garlic powder
2 teaspoons sugar
2½ pounds ripe tomatoes *or* 2 16-ounce
    cans tomatoes
4 cups chicken or beef broth
1 tablespoon lemon juice
1 teaspoon curry powder
2 bay leaves
2 peppercorns
¼ teaspoon thyme leaves
1 cup skim milk

Cook onion in oil until transparent. Add carrots, apple, and garlic, and cook, stirring until softened. Blend in sugar, tomatoes, broth, lemon juice, and seasonings. Cook over low heat until thickened or in electric slow cooker over medium heat for about 1½ hours. Strain out bay leaves and peppercorns. Puree in blender until smooth, and add 1 cup skim milk. Warm and serve immediately, or chill and serve cold.

Serves 8–10

Turkey Soup

3–4 pounds turkey wings or bony chicken
   pieces (backs, wings, and necks)
¼ cup pearl barley
⅓ cup navy or lima beans, soaked
   overnight
1 medium onion, chopped
¼ teaspoon basil
¼ teaspoon oregano
¼ teaspoon black pepper
½ teaspoon salt
1 cup frozen green peas
1 cup frozen corn
1 16-ounce can tomatoes

Cook turkey or chicken with barley, beans, onion, and
seasonings on low setting in electric slow cooker for 4 to
6 hours. Add frozen vegetables and tomatoes and cook
until done, about 30 minutes more.

Serves 8–10

Vegetable-Potato Soup

½ 20-ounce package frozen mixed
   vegetables
2 cups chicken broth
2 tablespoons instant or leftover mashed
   potatoes
1 cup milk
Grated Parmesan cheese (optional)

Cook the vegetables in the broth until just done. Add
potatoes and milk. Stir until thickened. Season with
freshly ground pepper. Garnish with grated Parmesan
cheese if desired.

Serves 3–4

VEGETABLES

Vegetables are our primary sources of vitamins A and C. Vitamin A is not affected by cooking unless vegetables are wilted before cooking or are overcooked. Vegetables that contain a lot of cellulose and are also high in vitamin A—such as mature beets, winter squash, carrots, green beans, sweet potatoes, and asparagus—yield more nutritional value cooked than raw. Cooking softens the cellulose and allows for greater absorption of the carotene, which is converted into vitamin A.

Vitamin C is easily altered to such an extent that the body cannot use it. It is destroyed by heat, air, and water, with the greatest destruction occurring when all three are combined. To decrease the losses, fruits and vegetables should be prepared as close to serving time as possible. The less they are cut up, the less they will be exposed to air and water. Whenever possible, serve vegetables and fruits raw, or at least cooked with as little water as possible and for as short a time as possible.

Learning to like crisp vegetables rather than mushy ones will add variety to your diet and also increase your nutrient intake. Stir-fried vegetables that are coated with oil and cooked for a very short period of time retain most of their vitamin C due to the decreased air exposure. Steaming vegetables or cooking them in minimum amounts of water in the microwave preserves vitamin C content. Pureeing vegetables when they are hot does not affect the vitamin A content, but does decrease the vitamin C content due to increased air exposure. Mashed or whipped potatoes are a poor source of vitamin C, whereas baked potatoes, cooked in their skins, are a good source.

Spicy Broccoli

2 cups steamed broccoli
1 cup cooked brown rice or noodles
2 large tomatoes, chopped
1 medium onion, chopped
3 tablespoons chopped fresh parsley
1 tablespoon oil
Dash of salt
¼ teaspoon black pepper
¼ teaspoon garlic powder

Combine all ingredients, cover, and refrigerate. Serve warm or cold.

Serves 6

Low-Calorie Baked Potatoes

4 baked potatoes
4 tablespoons plain low-fat yogurt
Freshly ground cumin

Split the potatoes and top each with 1 tablespoon plain low-fat yogurt. Sprinkle with freshly ground cumin.

Serves 4

Fresh Potato Salad

6 medium cooked potatoes, diced
1 cup celery, diced
1 medium onion, diced
1 cup mayonnaise or plain low-fat yogurt
1 medium cucumber, diced
1 teaspoon dill seed
Black pepper and salt to taste
Cherry tomatoes for garnish
Mint for garnish

Combine all ingredients except garnish, cover tightly, and chill. At serving time, garnish with cherry tomatoes and fresh mint.

Serves 6–8

Sweet Potato Bake

4 medium sweet potatoes, baked
1 16-ounce can pineapple chunks,
     including juice
2 teaspoons cinnamon
Pinch of cloves and ginger

Scoop potatoes out of shells, and combine with pineapple, pineapple juice, and spices. Place in buttered casserole dish and heat in oven until heated through, about 15 minutes.

Serves 4

Summer Squash Sauté

½ medium onion, diced
1 tablespoon oil
3 small zucchini, sliced
2 cups fresh corn, cut off the cob
½ teaspoon basil
¼ teaspoon thyme (use fresh if available)
Salt and pepper to taste

Brown the onion in a tablespoon of oil. Add zucchini, corn, and seasonings. Cook covered until tender, about 8 minutes.

Serves 6

Acorn Squash Delight

2 medium acorn squash
2 teaspoons brown sugar
1 16-ounce can unsweetened applesauce
2 tablespoons raisins or date pieces
Cinnamon, nutmeg, ground cloves to taste

Cut the squash in half and scoop out seeds. Place in casserole dish with 1 inch of water in the bottom. Fill the centers of the squash with brown sugar and applesauce. Top with raisins or dates and spices. Cover and bake in a 350°F oven until tender, about 30 minutes.

Serves 4–6

Quick Vegetable Medley

1 medium onion, chopped
2 teaspoons oil
1 green pepper, diced
1 16-ounce package frozen green beans
1 small zucchini, sliced
1 tablespoon chopped fresh parsley
5–6 tomatoes, chopped, *or* 1 16-ounce can
     peeled tomatoes
Dash each of onion, garlic powder, and
     black pepper
1 teaspoon oregano

Sauté onion in oil until clear, add green pepper, and cook 2 minutes. Add green beans, sliced zucchini, chopped parsley, tomatoes, and seasonings. Cook over low heat until tender, about 20 minutes.

Serves 6–8

SIDE DISHES
Herbed Barley Casserole

1 cup finely chopped celery
½ cup finely chopped scallions or onions
¼ cup oil
2 cups pearl barley
1 cup finely chopped parsley
4 cups chicken broth
1 cup slivered almonds

Sauté celery and scallions or onions in oil until just wilted. Add barley and brown it lightly. Stir in parsley and transfer mixture to a lightly buttered casserole with a lid. Pour 2 cups of broth over contents of casserole and bake covered for 30 minutes in a 350°F oven. Add the 2 remaining cups of broth and the nuts. Continue to bake until liquid is absorbed and barley is done, about 30 minutes longer. This dish freezes well for later use.

Serves 6–8

Posole

Posole is corn that has been treated to remove the bran and then dried. It is available in the Spanish food section of the grocery store.

1 cup posole
3 cups water
½ teaspoon salt
¼ teaspoon black pepper
2 teaspoons vegetable oil

Soak the posole for 1 hour in the water. Add the seasonings and cook the posole in a 350°F oven for 45 minutes. Stir in 2 teaspoons vegetable oil before serving.
Note: Other seasonings you might enjoy are green or red chili or sage.

Serves 4–6

Brown Rice

1 cup brown rice
3 cups water
½ teaspoon salt

Place all ingredients in a covered casserole dish and cook in a 350°F oven for 30 to 40 minutes. Cooked this way, rice does not have to be watched constantly. If it should cook dry, the rice will toast rather than burn.

Makes 3 cups

Brown Rice with Vegetables

1 small onion
2 stalks celery, diced
2 tablespoons oil
1 cup frozen or fresh peas *or* 1 medium
    zucchini, sliced
2 cups cooked brown rice
2 cups chicken broth
⅓ cup slivered almonds

Cook onion and celery in oil until limp. Place in casserole with vegetables, brown rice, chicken broth, and slivered almonds. Bake at 350°F for 30 minutes.

Serves 4–6

Oriental Fried Rice

1 tablespoon peanut or sesame oil
1 stalk broccoli, cut into medium-size
    pieces
¼ small head cauliflower, cut into
    medium-size pieces
2 medium carrots, diced
1 small zucchini
1 medium onion, diced
1 large stalk celery, diced
4 cups cooked brown rice
Pinch of cloves and garlic powder
¼ teaspoon black pepper
Salt to taste
Soy sauce (optional)
Tofu (optional)

Heat the oil in a heavy pan; stir-fry the broccoli, cauliflower, and carrots for 3 minutes; add the other vegetables, and continue cooking for 3 minutes. Stir in rice and seasonings and cook until heated through. Tofu may be added to this dish to make a complete protein.

Serves 6–8

ENTREES
Herbed and Spiced Beef

3 pounds (bone in) chuck roast
1 large onion, chopped
2 cups beef broth
2 tablespoons lemon juice
2 bay leaves
1 teaspoon thyme leaves
5 each whole cloves, allspice berries
3 peppercorns

Place all ingredients in electric slow cooker and cook on low setting overnight. Cool and skim off fat. Warm and serve with rice, noodles, or baked potatoes.

Serves 6–8

Spanish Brown Rice with Beef

½ pound lean ground beef
1 20-ounce package frozen mixed
   vegetables
1 16-ounce can tomatoes *or* 3 large
   tomatoes, peeled and pureed
½ teaspoon oregano
½ teaspoon chili powder
¼ teaspoon salt
¼ teaspoon garlic powder
Freshly ground black pepper *or* ¼
   teaspoon Mr. Pepper
3 cups cooked brown rice

Brown meat, breaking it into pieces and stirring for about 5 minutes. Add all other ingredients and continue cooking, stirring occasionally until heated through (about 10 minutes). Serve immediately.

Serves 4

Tenderfoot Chili

2 pounds lean ground beef
1 medium onion, chopped fine
2 cloves garlic, chopped fine
1 small carrot, diced
1 rib celery, diced
1 sweet green pepper, diced
2 tablespoons chili powder
2 tablespoons paprika
1 teaspoon leaf basil
½ teaspoon ground cumin
½ teaspoon ground coriander
1 16-ounce can tomatoes *or* 5 medium
    fresh tomatoes, diced
2 tablespoons tomato paste
1 16-ounce can or 2 cups cooked kidney or
    pinto beans
¼ teaspoon salt

Sauté beef. Add onion, garlic, carrot, celery, and green pepper, and cook until onion is transparent. Add chili powder, paprika, basil, cumin, coriander, tomatoes, and tomato paste. Bring to boil and simmer, stirring occasionally, for 1½ hours, or cook in electric slow cooker on medium setting. Add beans and salt, cook until heated through, and serve.

Serves 6–8

Herbed Pork Chops

1 tablespoon rosemary
1 tablespoon sage
2 teaspoons diced garlic *or* dash of garlic
  powder
2 1-inch pork chops
2 tablespoons oil
Juice of 1 lemon
½ cup chicken broth or water

Mix together rosemary, sage, and garlic, and press firmly into both sides of pork chops. Brown pork chops on both sides in oil over medium heat. Sprinkle pork chops with half the lemon juice, add chicken broth or water, and after bringing this mixture to a rapid boil, lower the heat to medium and braise for 45 minutes. Remove chops to a warm plate. Add remaining lemon juice to the cooking liquid and pour over the meat or accompanying rice, noodles, or potatoes.

Serves 2

Apricot Chicken

8 chicken thighs or drumsticks
¼ cup no-sugar apricot jam
2 tablespoons lemon juice

Broil the chicken and baste with a mixture of the jam and lemon juice as it cooks.

Serves 4

Baked Chicken with Tomatoes

4–6 chicken breasts
1 large onion, diced
1 16-ounce can whole peeled tomatoes *or*
  1–3 fresh tomatoes
Fresh parsley, chopped
2 tablespoons lemon juice

Place chicken breasts in casserole, and cover with onion, tomatoes, parsley, and lemon juice. Cover and bake at 350°F for 1 hour. Remove cover for last few minutes of baking so chicken will brown.

Serves 4–6

Baked Chicken with Vegetables

4–6 chicken breasts or pieces
1 large onion, diced
4 stalks celery, diced
4–6 carrots, scraped and diced
Fresh parsley, chopped
Pinch each of onion, garlic powder, and
    black pepper
¼ teaspoon dill weed
½ teaspoon oregano or Italian seasoning
¼ cup lemon juice
1–2 small zucchini, sliced

Cook chicken in large covered casserole along with all the other ingredients, except zucchini, at 350°F for about 30 minutes. Add zucchini and continue cooking for 30 minutes more.

Serves 4–6

Chicken, Spanish Style

8 chicken thighs or drumsticks
1 teaspoon chili powder *or* 2 teaspoons
    canned green chili
1 medium onion, chopped
½ cup carrot, diced
1 16-ounce can tomatoes
1 cup frozen green peas
3 cups cooked brown rice

Bake the chicken with chili powder and onion in a casserole dish with a small amount of water in a 350°F oven, until about half done (30 minutes). Add vegetables and brown rice and continue cooking for 20 minutes more.

Serves 4

Curried Chicken Salad

2 tablespoons curry powder
½ cup mayonnaise or plain low-fat yogurt
2 cups cooked, diced chicken (canned may
    be used)
1½ cups celery, diced
½ cup raisins
1 red or green pepper, diced
1 orange, peeled and cut into bite-size
    pieces
½ cup chopped or slivered almonds
1 cup green or red seedless grapes
Lettuce to make beds for salad

Add curry powder to mayonnaise or yogurt and mix together. Pour over other ingredients except lettuce, combine, and refrigerate for at least 1 hour before serving on beds of lettuce.

Serves 4

Italian Oven-Fried Chicken

8 drumsticks or thighs
Italian Coating Mix (recipe follows)

Rinse chicken and roll in the coating mix. Place in a buttered casserole dish and bake in 350°F oven for about 45 minutes.

Serves 4

Italian Coating Mix

1 cup crushed whole-wheat crackers or
    whole-wheat bread crumbs
1½ tablespoons instant diced onions
2 teaspoons oregano
½ teaspoon marjoram
¼ teaspoon black pepper
¼ teaspoon dry mustard
⅛ teaspoon cayenne pepper
½ teaspoon salt

Combine all ingredients in a blender or food processor. Whirl until crackers or bread are finely crumbled. Store in the refrigerator.

Baked Fish

1 pound fresh or thawed frozen salmon,
    red snapper, perch, or cod
Dash of black pepper, garlic, and onion
    powder
1 tablespoon lemon juice

Place fish in lightly buttered baking dish. Sprinkle with seasonings and lemon juice. Cover and bake for approximately 20 minutes. Uncover for the last 5 minutes so it will brown. Some of the homemade seasoning blends also work well with fish.

Serves 3–4

Fish with Tomatoes

1 12-ounce package cod, perch, sole, or
    turbot, defrosted
2 tomatoes, chopped
Fresh parsley, chopped
½ teaspoon basil
½ teaspoon dill weed
Dash each of black pepper, onion powder,
    and garlic powder
2 tablespoons lemon juice

Place fish in lightly buttered baking dish, add tomatoes
and seasonings. Cover and bake at 350°F for about 20
minutes. If frozen fish is used, allow 45 minutes to 1
hour of baking time.

Serves 3–4

Eggplant Casserole

1 large eggplant, pared and cut into ½-
    inch slices
1 tablespoon safflower oil
1 small onion, chopped
1 small garlic clove, cut in half
1 stalk celery, diced
1 16-ounce can tomatoes
2 teaspoons basil
1 teaspoon oregano
⅛ teaspoon black pepper
3 ounces egg noodles, cooked
¼ cup cottage cheese
8 ounces shredded low-fat cheese

Cook the eggplant in the oil. Add onion, garlic, celery,
tomatoes, and seasonings, and cook 5 minutes. Layer
the noodles, vegetable mixture, and cottage cheese.
Sprinkle with shredded cheese and bake at 350°F for
30 minutes.

Serves 3–4

Guacamole Chalupas

2 large ripe avocados, halved, pitted, and
    peeled
1 tablespoon lemon juice
1 small onion, chopped fine
5 medium ripe tomatoes, chopped coarse
½ teaspoon salt
½ teaspoon black pepper
12 corn tortillas (see Index) or 1 package
    corn tortillas
1 tablespoon oil
2 cups shredded leaf lettuce
1½ cups shredded cheese

Prepare guacamole by mashing avocados and mixing with lemon juice, onion, one tomato, salt, and pepper. Cover and refrigerate for at least 1 hour. Brown tortillas in oil. Place each tortilla in the center of a plate, top with ⅓ cup guacamole, spreading it to within ½ inch of the border. Top each tortilla with lettuce, remaining chopped tomato, and cheese. To eat, they may be rolled or folded in half like a taco.

Serves 6

BROWN BAG LUNCHES
Spicy Brisket

3 pounds beef brisket
4 peppercorns
2 bay leaves
½ teaspoon salt
Pinch of ground cloves
1 16-ounce can tomatoes

Place all ingredients in electric slow cooker with enough water to cover and cook overnight. The brisket makes good beef sandwiches. The broth can be used in other recipes calling for beef broth or frozen for later use.

Peanut Butter Sandwiches

2 slices whole-wheat bread
2 tablespoons peanut butter
1 tablespoon grated carrot
Raisins
Ground cinnamon

Spread 1 slice whole-wheat bread with peanut butter. Top with 1 tablespoon of grated carrot and a few raisins. Sprinkle with cinnamon. Top with remaining slice of bread.

Serves 1

Chicken Salad

1 6-ounce can chicken, diced
1 tablespoon cashews or almonds
20 fresh grapes, if in season, *or* 1 apple, diced
2 ribs celery, diced
2 tablespoons plain low-fat yogurt
Salt and pepper to taste

Combine all ingredients. May be served on lettuce leaves or used in sandwiches. Refrigerate until serving time.

Makes 2 cups

BREADS
Biscuits from Mix

¼ cup oil or shortening
2½ cups Whole-Grain Baking Mix (see Index)
¾ cup milk

Cut oil into the baking mix with pastry blender until the mixture resembles coarse cornmeal. Add milk gradually and stir until mixture forms ball in the bowl. Roll ½ inch thick and cut into rounds. Place on ungreased baking sheet and bake at 400°F for 10–15 minutes.

Makes 12–18

Biscuits from Scratch

2 cups whole-wheat flour
½ teaspoon salt
1 tablespoon baking powder
¼ cup shortening
¾ cup milk

Mix dry ingredients. Cut shortening into flour mixture until it resembles coarse cornmeal. Add milk to make a stiff dough. Knead lightly on floured bread board. Roll to ½-inch thickness and cut into rounds. Bake at 400°F for 10 minutes.

Makes 12–18

Bran Muffins

½ cup millers' or oat bran
1½ cups whole-wheat flour
2 tablespoons molasses
3 tablespoons oil
½ teaspoon salt
2 teaspoons baking powder
1 egg
¾ cup milk

Mix all ingredients and spoon into buttered muffin tins. Bake at 350°F for about 20 minutes.

Makes 1 dozen

Chapatis (East Indian Bread)

2 cups whole-wheat flour
1 tablespoon oil
½ teaspoon salt
¾–1 cup warm water

Mix all ingredients, adding more water if necessary to form soft dough. Let stand for 5 minutes. Turn dough onto lightly greased surface and let stand at room temperature for 1 hour. Divide dough into 16 equal parts. Roll out each part into a thin circle 6 to 8 inches in diameter on a lightly floured surface. Cook in lightly greased heavy skillet until brown.

Makes 16

Corn Bread

1½ cups cornmeal
½ cup whole-wheat flour
¼ cup powdered milk
½ teaspoon salt
2 teaspoons baking powder
2 teaspoons sugar
1 egg
2 tablespoons oil
1½ cups milk

Mix dry ingredients. Add egg, oil, and milk, and mix. Pour into 8-inch square baking pan and bake at 350°F for 20 to 30 minutes.

Makes 16 squares

Corn Tortillas

2 cups masa harina
1¼–1½ cups warm water

Mix ingredients until stiff dough is formed. Turn onto lightly greased surface and divide into 12 equal parts. Shape into smooth balls. Place between two pieces of waxed paper and flatten into a circle, or place in tortilla press and press down firmly. Cook on lightly greased hot griddle or in a heavy skillet until lightly browned.

Makes 12

Fruit Nut Bread

1½ cups whole-wheat pastry flour
½ teaspoon salt
1 tablespoon baking powder
½ cup nuts
¼ cup sugar, honey, or molasses
1 egg
3 tablespoons oil
½ cup milk
½ cup dried apricots, soaked

Mix dry ingredients together. Blend in liquid ingredients and apricots. Pour into greased loaf pan. Bake at 350°F for about 45 minutes. May also be baked in muffin tins.

Note: For the dried apricots, you may substitute one of the following: 1½ cups chopped dates, 1 cup cranberries and 2 tablespoons orange juice concentrate, 1 cup (2–3) mashed ripe bananas, or 1 cup applesauce and 2 teaspoons cinnamon, with a pinch of nutmeg and ground cloves.

Makes two small loaves

Griddle Cakes from Scratch

2 cups whole-wheat flour
1 tablespoon baking powder
½ teaspoon salt
1 tablespoon sugar, honey, or molasses
1 egg
2 tablespoons oil
1½ cups milk

Mix dry ingredients together, add liquids, and stir until smooth. Bake on lightly greased griddle, turning only once when top shows bubbles all over. If thicker cakes are desired, reduce amount of milk in recipe.

Makes about 24 3-inch cakes

Honey Graham Crackers

1 cup whole-wheat flour
1 cup white flour
¼ cup brown sugar
1 teaspoon baking powder
½ teaspoon salt
½ cup Butter-Not
¼ cup honey
¼ cup oil
3 tablespoons cold water

Mix dry ingredients and liquids separately, then blend together to form dough. Divide the dough in half, place each half on an ungreased baking sheet, and roll to flatten, dusting lightly with flour to avoid sticking. Score with a knife to make 2-inch squares. Prick with a fork. Bake at 425°F for 8 to 10 minutes. Remove from oven and cut apart while hot.

Makes 3 dozen

Hot Cakes from Mix

3 tablespoons oil
1 egg
2½ cups milk or water
3 cups whole-grain Baking Mix (see
Index) *or* 2 cups mix and 1 cup
buckwheat flour

Mix oil, egg, and milk or water. Add to Baking Mix and stir until well combined. Cook on lightly greased griddle.

Makes 10 4-inch cakes

Irish Soda Bread

4 cups whole-wheat flour
½ cup sugar
1 teaspoon salt
2 teaspoons baking powder
½ cup safflower oil
1¾ cups milk
¼ cup raisins

Sift dry ingredients together. Add oil, milk, and raisins. Knead, adding more flour if needed. Divide into two loaves. Put into buttered loaf pans and bake at 350°F for 30 to 40 minutes.

Makes 2 loaves

Mountain Bread

4 cups whole-wheat flour
1 cup water
4 tablespoons brown sugar
½ cup honey
⅓ cup wheat germ
¼ cup sesame seeds
¼ cup molasses
3 tablespoons powdered milk
2 teaspoons baking powder
½ teaspoon salt

Mix all ingredients until smooth. Pour into well-greased 8-inch square baking pan and bake at 300°F for 1 hour, or until bread pulls away from sides of pan. Cut into squares and let stand overnight to dry before wrapping, or serve immediately.

Makes 16 squares

Muffins from Mix

3 tablespoons oil
1 egg
1 tablespoon honey or molasses if
    additional sweetness is desired
1 cup milk or water
2½ cups Whole-Grain Baking Mix (see
    Index)

Mix oil, egg, honey, and milk or water, and add to baking mix. Stir 20 times. Bake in well-greased muffin tins at 400°F for about 20 minutes.

Makes 12

Oat Crackers

1 cup oat flour (grind oatmeal in a
    blender)
¼ cup whole-wheat flour
2 teaspoons baking powder
¼ teaspoon salt
1 egg
2 tablespoons oil
3 tablespoons water or milk

Combine all ingredients and mix thoroughly. Place on greased cookie sheet and roll to desired thickness. Cut into squares. Bake at 350°F for about 20 minutes. Watch carefully to avoid burning the edges. Store in refrigerator to keep oil from changing flavor.

Makes 24

Popovers

1 egg
½ teaspoon salt
½ cup milk
½ cup whole-wheat pastry flour

Butter and heat muffin tins for 12, then prepare the batter. Blend the egg, salt, and milk in a blender. Gradually add the flour. Pour into buttered, hot muffin tins. Bake at 350°F for 25 minutes.

Note: The secret to success lies in preheating the muffin tins.

Makes 9–12

Pumpernickel Bread

3½ cups milk
2 packages yeast
2 tablespoons oil
1½ tablespoons salt
2 cups mashed potatoes
¼ cup dark molasses
9 cups whole-wheat flour
3 cups rye flour
1 cup millers' bran or oat bran
Caraway seed (optional)

Heat milk until it feels warm to the touch. Add yeast, oil, salt, potatoes, molasses, and enough whole-wheat flour to make a batter. Beat with mixer until thick. Add rye flour and bran, and mix. Knead and allow to rise until double in bulk. Divide into three loaves. Place in buttered loaf pans. Sprinkle with caraway seeds if desired. Allow to rise slightly. Bake in 350°F oven for 40 minutes.

Makes 3 loaves

Sesame Crackers

2 cups whole-wheat pastry flour
1 teaspoon baking powder
½ teaspoon salt
⅔ cup water
⅓ cup oil
1 egg white beaten with 2 tablespoons
    water
4 tablespoons sesame seeds

Mix all ingredients except egg white and sesame seeds in bowl to make dough. Divide in half, cover, and let stand 10 to 20 minutes. Place each half of the dough on a lightly oiled cookie sheet. Roll out to desired thickness, score into 2-inch squares and prick with a fork. Brush with beaten egg white and sprinkle with sesame seeds. Bake in 400°F oven about 8 minutes. For herb crackers, add 1½ teaspoons mixed salad herbs or Italian herbs to the mixture.

Makes 3 dozen

Southern Corn Bread Dressing

½ medium onion, chopped
1 cup celery, diced
¼ cup drippings from poultry or vegetable oil
4 cups crumbled corn bread
4 cups crumbled biscuits
1 teaspoon salt
¼ teaspoon pepper
½ teaspoon poultry seasoning
1 egg
1 cup stock *or* bouillon cube in one cup water

Cook onion and celery in drippings or oil until tender. Add corn bread and biscuits, salt, pepper, and poultry seasoning. Place in baking dish. Beat egg slightly and add to stock. Pour over dressing and mix. Bake 30–45 minutes at 350°F. May also be placed in roasting pan around a turkey or chicken for the last hour of cooking so that juices from meat soak into it.

Makes enough to stuff a 10-pound turkey or two medium-sized chickens

Waffles from Scratch

2 cups whole-wheat flour
1 tablespoon baking powder
½ teaspoon salt
1 tablespoon sugar, honey, or molasses
3 egg yolks
1½ cups milk
⅓ cup oil
3 egg whites, beaten stiff

Mix all ingredients except egg whites to make a smooth batter. Fold in the egg whites. Bake on ungreased waffle iron.

Makes 6–8

Whole-Grain Baking Mix

12 cups whole-wheat flour
2 cups powdered milk
6 tablespoons baking powder
2½ teaspoons salt
½ cup sugar

Sift all ingredients together and store in covered container.
   Note: This mix is used in several Breads and Desserts recipes.

Whole-Wheat Date Nut Bread

2 cups whole-wheat pastry flour
½ teaspoon salt
1 tablespoon baking powder
3 tablespoons sugar, honey, or molasses
1 egg
3 tablespoons oil
1 cup milk
⅔ cup chopped dates
⅓ cup nuts

Mix flour, salt, baking powder, and sugar; add liquids, stirring to make a smooth batter. Blend in dates and nuts. Pour into two greased loaf pans. Bake at 350°F for approximately 45 minutes.

Makes two small loaves

Whole-Wheat Tortillas

2 cups whole-wheat flour
¼ cup lard, butter, or shortening
½ teaspoon salt
½–¾ cup warm water
2 teaspoons baking powder

Mix all ingredients thoroughly. Turn onto lightly greased surface. Divide into 12 equal parts. Shape each into a smooth ball. Roll out each ball into a circle approximately 8 inches in diameter on lightly floured surface. Cook on lightly greased griddle or in heavy skillet until browned on both sides.

Makes 12

DESSERTS

No-Sugar Baked Apples

4 apples (Golden Delicious, McIntosh,
    Cortland, etc.)
Dash each of cinnamon, cloves, and
    nutmeg
Raisins *or* chopped dates
Water

Wash and core apples. Sprinkle centers with cinnamon, cloves, and nutmeg. Place in lightly buttered baking dish. Stuff the centers with raisins or chopped dates. Add 1 tablespoon water and bake in covered container at 350°F for about 30 minutes.

Serves 4

Apricot-Oatmeal Squares

1 tablespoon lemon juice
11 ounces dried apricots
1 cup and 2 tablespoons water
2¼ cups oat flour (grind oatmeal in a
     blender, ¾ cup at a time)
1½ teaspoons cinnamon
¼ teaspoon ground ginger
¼ cup honey
1 cup oil

Combine lemon juice, apricots, and water in a saucepan, and heat thoroughly to make sauce. Set aside. Combine oat flour, cinnamon, ginger, honey, and oil. Mixture should be slightly crumbly. Press half the mixture into oiled 9-inch pan. Cover with apricot sauce, and spread remaining oat mixture on top. Bake at 350°F for 30 minutes or until light brown. Refrigerate overnight for easier cutting.

Makes about 16 squares

Gingerbread Sculpture

This is a popular holiday recipe for young children because they can mold the dough into anything they want, bake it, and then eat it.

⅓ cup oil
1 cup brown sugar
1½ cups dark molasses
⅔ cup water
6 cups whole wheat flour
1 tablespoon baking powder
½ teaspoon salt
½ teaspoon cinnamon
¼ teaspoon ground ginger

Mix all ingredients together. The dough should be stiff. Shapes can be molded and decorated with nuts and raisins, or the dough can be rolled and cut into shapes. Bake at 350°F for 7 to 10 minutes.

Makes 4 dozen

Oatmeal Cookies from Mix

> 1 cup rolled oats
> 2¾ cups Whole-Grain Baking Mix (see Index)
> ½ cup of any or all of the following: coconut, raisins, nuts, or sunflower seeds
> 1 egg
> ¾ cup honey *or* 1 cup sugar and ¼ cup water
> ½ cup oil

Combine oats, Baking Mix, and coconut, raisins, nuts, or seeds. Add remaining ingredients and stir until well mixed. Drop by the teaspoon on a greased cookie sheet. Allow room between cookies for spreading. Bake at 350°F for 10 to 15 minutes.

Makes 4 dozen

Fortified Oatmeal Cookies

1 cup sugar
1 tablespoon baking powder
1 cup whole-wheat flour
3 cups oatmeal
¼ cup powdered milk
1 cup raisins
1 cup nuts or sunflower seeds (optional)
½ cup oil
2 eggs
6 tablespoons dark molasses
Milk or water

Mix all the dry ingredients together. Add oil, eggs, molasses, and enough milk or water to make a thick dough. Drop by the teaspoon on a buttered cookie sheet or spread on cookie sheet to make bars. Bake at 350°F for 10 to 12 minutes.

Note: Despite the sugar content of this recipe, the amount of available sugar is less than in most similar recipes. This is the dietitian's answer to granola bars, which are excessively high in sugar.

Makes about 3 dozen

Peanut Butter Cookies from Mix

3 cups Whole-Grain Baking Mix (see Index)
½ cup oil
¾ cup honey *or* 1 cup sugar and ¼ cup liquid
1 egg
½ cup peanut butter

Mix all ingredients together. Drop on ungreased cookie sheet and press with a fork to flatten. Bake at 350°F for about 10 minutes.

Makes 4 dozen

Pie Crust

1 cup whole-wheat pastry flour
½ teaspoon salt
⅓ cup shortening
2–3 tablespoons water

Mix flour and salt. Cut shortening in until it is the size of peas. Add water to make a stiff dough. Knead lightly on floured board. Roll until quite thin. Place in pie tin and shape as desired. For lower-calorie desserts that seem special, pie crust can be cut into small, fancy shapes with cookie cutters, sprinkled with cinnamon, and baked for use as topping on fresh fruit desserts.

Makes 1 crust

Non-Wheat Pie Crust

1 tablespoon butter or oil
1½ cups cooked brown rice
Mix butter or oil and rice. Press into a pie tin and toast lightly before putting in pie filling.

Makes 1 crust

Pineapple-Apricot Yogurt

1 15-ounce can crushed pineapple in juice
1 16-ounce can apricots in juice
1 envelope plain gelatin
¼ cup honey
16 ounces plain yogurt
1 teaspoon vanilla

Drain juice from canned fruits into a saucepan, and sprinkle gelatin over juice. Let stand 5 minutes. Place saucepan over very low heat, stirring constantly until gelatin dissolves. Remove from heat and stir in honey. Cool. Puree apricots in blender and combine apricots, pineapple, yogurt, and vanilla with gelatin mixture. Cool in refrigerator or freeze until mushy, and beat with electric mixer until smooth. Frozen, this mixture can be cut into squares and put between graham crackers to make an ice cream–type sandwich.

Serves 4–6

Pumpkin Pie

1 16-ounce can pumpkin
½ cup sugar
1 teaspoon cinnamon
½ teaspoon each ground ginger, allspice,
    and cloves
1 cup apple juice
2 eggs, beaten
Prepared pie crust (optional)

Mix all ingredients together. Pour into lightly oiled pie plate or pie crust. Bake at 350°F for 45 minutes, or until knife inserted in center comes out clean.

Makes 1 pie

Rice Pudding

¼ cup sugar
¼ teaspoon salt
1½ cups cooked brown rice
1 teaspoon vanilla
1 cup raisins, plumped in water and
    drained
1 tablespoon grated orange rind
1 teaspoon grated lemon rind
3½ cups milk
3 eggs

Mix all ingredients except milk and eggs; pour into greased 2-quart casserole. Blend milk and eggs and pour over other ingredients. Set the casserole in a dish of water in the oven to prevent the eggs from curdling. Bake at 350°F for about 1 hour. Serve warm or chilled.

Serves 6–8

Sautéed Apple and Nut Dessert

1 tablespoon butter
2 tablespoons oil
2 apples, cut into ½-inch slices
1–2 tablespoons lemon juice
3 tablespoons chopped nuts

Heat the butter and oil in a skillet until bubbling but not browned. Add sliced apples and heat, stirring a bit. Turn the apples over after about 2 minutes. Sprinkle with lemon juice and nuts. Continue stirring for another minute. Serve warm.

Serves 4

Sautéed Bananas

2 ripe, firm bananas
2–3 teaspoons butter
1 tablespoon fresh lime juice
Dash of cinnamon, ginger, or nutmeg
    (optional)

Melt the butter in a skillet. Peel and split the bananas lengthwise. Sauté them for 1 minute over low heat. Pour lime juice over the bananas, turn them over carefully, and sauté for another minute; sprinkle with spices if desired. Serve warm.

Serves 2–4

SAUCES AND SANDWICH SPREADS

Chutney

3 tart apples, diced
½ cup chopped onion
1 teaspoon finely minced garlic
½ cup brown sugar
¼ cup lemon or lime juice
¾ teaspoon ground allspice
¾ teaspoon ground cloves
¾ teaspoon ground ginger
¼ teaspoon black pepper
¾ cup crushed pineapple
1 cup raisins
¼ cup chopped dates, prunes, or black figs

Mix all ingredients except dried fruit in saucepan. Bring to boil and simmer for 10 minutes. Add dried fruit, return to boil, and cook for 20 minutes. Store in refrigerator. Use as condiment with meat and poultry.

Fresh Green Chutney

1 cup minced fresh cilantro, tightly
    packed
½ cup minced fresh mint, tightly packed
⅓ cup lemon juice
1 fresh mild or hot green chili, diced, *or* 1
    small can diced green chili
2 cloves garlic, minced
1 tablespoon grated fresh ginger
1 tablespoon oil
¼ teaspoon salt

Mix all ingredients together in blender or food processor and chill. May be prepared a day ahead of time and refrigerated. Serve with beef or lamb.

Blender Mayonnaise

1 egg
1 teaspoon dry mustard
Scant ½ teaspoon salt
Dash cayenne pepper
1¼ cups salad oil
2 tablespoons lemon juice

Place egg, mustard, salt, cayenne, and ¼ cup oil in blender. Blend at high speed until completely mixed. Add the lemon juice slowly. With blender running, take off center of cover and slowly pour in oil, 2 tablespoons at a time, until the mixture is thick. It might be necessary to turn off the blender and scrape down the sides occasionally. Vinegar may be used instead of the lemon juice. If you live alone or do not use mayonnaise often, make half the recipe. In order to halve the egg, beat it, measure, and divide into equal parts. Add the extra to some other dish.

Homemade Mustard

¼ cup mustard seeds
6 tablespoons dry mustard
1 tablespoon turmeric (optional)
1 teaspoon dried tarragon
1¼ cups boiling water
½ cup lemon juice
1 tablespoon vegetable oil
¼ cup sugar
½ cup finely chopped onion
2 teaspoons finely minced garlic
¼ teaspoon ground allspice
¼ teaspoon ground cinnamon
¼ teaspoon ground cloves

Combine mustard seeds, dry mustard, turmeric if desired, tarragon, and boiling water in bowl. Let stand 1 hour. Combine remaining ingredients in saucepan, bring to boil, and simmer for 5 minutes. Blend the two mixtures in blender for 2 minutes. Cook in top of double boiler for about 5 minutes, or until thickened.

Sweet-and-Sour Sauce

¾ cup water
½ cup sugar
¼ cup vinegar
1 tablespoon cornstarch
¼ cup tomato sauce
Dash each of black pepper, cloves, dry
    mustard, and garlic powder
1 tablespoon finely chopped fresh ginger
    (optional)
¼ cup finely chopped onion

Combine water, sugar, vinegar, and cornstarch in a saucepan. Stir until cornstarch is dissolved. Add the remaining ingredients and cook over low heat until thickened. Store in refrigerator.

Fruited Sweet and Sour Sauce

¼ cup frozen pineapple juice concentrate
3 tablespoons lemon juice
Dash each of black pepper, cloves, dry
    mustard, and garlic powder
¼ cup finely chopped onion

Combine all ingredients. Store in refrigerator. Serve with poultry or meat.

Yogurt Sauce

1 cup lemon mayonnaise *or* 1 cup plain
    yogurt or half of each
½ teaspoon ground coriander
Pinch of salt
¼ teaspoon turmeric (optional)
¼ teaspoon paprika
Pinch of hot green chili

Blend all ingredients and chill. May be prepared a day ahead of time and refrigerated.

SNACKS

Frozen Bananas

Cut firm ripe bananas in half and put on a Popsicle stick if desired. These may be frozen and then eaten as Popsicles or coated with melted chocolate for additional sweetness.

Tiger Candy

1 cup crunchy peanut butter
½ cup instant powdered milk
¼ cup honey
2 tablespoons raisins
Grated coconut (optional)

Mix all ingredients with hands. If the mixture is too dry, add a small amount of liquid milk. If it is too wet, add a small amount of powdered milk. Roll into small balls and chill. May be rolled in coconut, if desired.

Home-Roasted Peanuts

1 pound raw Spanish or Virginia peanuts

Spread peanuts evenly on a cookie sheet with sides. Place in low (250°F) oven for 10 minutes. Stir if necessary. Turn oven off and leave peanuts in oven until skins are lightly browned.

Pepitas

1 tablespoon oil
1 pound raw pumpkin seeds
Combine oil and pumpkin seeds and heat in heavy skillet, stirring constantly, until the seeds pop and the halves of the seeds separate. Season with salt or herbs.

Frozen Pops

2 cups fruit juice
1 teaspoon plain gelatin, dissolved in
    warm water

Mix the gelatin and juice, pour into Popsicle containers or ice-cube trays. If ice cube trays are used, insert toothpicks when the mixture is partially frozen. Freeze until firm.

Frozen Grape Treats

Seedless green or red grapes, washed and
removed from stems

Spread grapes on cookie sheet and freeze. Place in
plastic bag for snacking. These make sweet snacks that
are low in calories and that seem to be popular with
everyone.

Raw Vegetable Dip

1 cup plain low-fat yogurt
1 tablespoon chopped chives or other
    herbs
Pinch of salt
2 tablespoons mayonnaise
Raw vegetables to dip

Mix all ingredients and chill. Serve with assorted raw
vegetables as dippers.
  Note: Other seasonings that could be used are dill,
oregano, thyme, onion powder, garlic powder, Tabasco
sauce, or salad herb blends.

SNACK ITEMS TO KEEP ON HAND
Whole-wheat crackers
Rye Crisps
Rice cakes, squares, and chips
Lightly roasted peanuts
Raw almonds and sunflower seeds
Peanut or almond butter
Low-fat cheeses
Low-salt corn chips
Dried and fresh fruit
Milk
Yogurt
Raw vegetables
Popcorn
Whole-wheat and corn tortillas (these keep
    well frozen and are easily separated)

Index